The Consumer Handbook on Hearing Loss and Hearing Aids A Bridge to Healing

FOURTH EDITION

Richard E. Carmen, AuD
Editor

Auricle Ink Publishers
Sedona

Library of Congress Cataloging-in-Publication Data

The consumer handbook on hearing loss and hearing aids : a bridge to healing
/ Richard E. Carmen, AuD, editor. -- Fourth edition.
    pages cm
 Includes bibliographical references and index.
  ISBN 978-0-9825785-5-1 (softcover : alk. paper) -- ISBN 978-0-9825785-6-8
(hardcover :alk. paper)
1. Deafness--Popular works. 2. Hearing disorders--Popular works. 3. Hearing
aids--Popular works. I. Carmen, Richard E., editor of compilation.
  RF291.35.C665 2014
  617.8--dc23

                        2013029752

©2014
Auricle Ink Publishers

ISBN: 978-0-9825785-5-1 (Soft Cover)
Printing 10 9 8 7 6 5 4 3 2 1
ISBN: 978-0-9825785-6-8 (Hard Cover)
Printing 10 9 8 7 6 5 4 3 2 1

Cover concept and development by Bradley Peterson
Unique Graphic Art, Tucson, AZ

This book is available at special discount when ordered in bulk.
Contact the publisher for more information.

Auricle Ink Publishers
P. O. Box 20607
Sedona AZ 86341
(928) 284-0860
www.hearingproblems.com
Email: AIP@hearingproblems.com

Dedicated to you
transforming
hope into action.

CONTENTS

FOREWORD

I recently retired from the field of audiology after forty years of testing hearing, dispensing hearing aids, and providing group aural rehabilitation/counseling sessions for adults with hearing loss. The last twenty years were spent at Mayo Clinic where I was director of the Mayo Hearing Aid Clinic and had a very active adult aural rehabilitation program. I have spent thousands of hours saying to patients many of the things that are mentioned and discussed in this excellent book.

It had been ten years since I read an earlier edition of Dr. Carmen's book, and I thought that I probably could write a Foreword without reading this new edition. However, with my expanded spare time in retirement, I decided to read it in its entirety and I am very glad I did. Why? Because I now have a hearing loss and I have not done anything about it! In spite of knowing virtually everything in the book from my professional audiologist viewpoint and providing the information and counseling to patients for years, I found myself reading the book as a 64-year-old guy with a hearing loss who has been putting off doing anything about it. To say the least this book provided me with some interesting insights.

So what did I find particularly meaningful and enlightening in the book? The two chapters by Sergei Kochkin are a great summary of his years of market studies that have shed light on the benefits of hearing aids and their impact on quality of life. It reminded me that hearing aids really do help—who wouldn't want to improve relationships at home, feelings about yourself, and have a better overall quality of life? His list of realistic expectations for hearing aids is excellent and important knowledge for the consumer.

My friend Robert Sweetow's chapter on hearing aid technology was also a great overview. Since 'information is power,' consumers will be empowered after learning about hearing aid circuitry options. I liked his wise piece of advice when he stated that to be successful with hearing aids, one must ". . . be patient with yourself, have a sense of humor, and maintain realistic expectations."

The more informational oriented chapters in this book, such as those by Robert Sweetow, Kris English (the audiogram), David Myers (telecoils), Robert Sandlin (professionals in hearing care), and Grant Searchfield (tinnitus) are quite good and should be a valuable resource to the reader with hearing loss. The chapters that I liked the most, and from which readers will greatly benefit, were those that dealt with emotional aspects of hearing loss and/or provided a framework for positive actions that can be taken. These include the chapters by James Maurer (it's your brain that hears and it's pliable; be positive and active physically and mentally), Richard Carmen (acknowledge your hearing loss, be open to change, you're not alone, do something about it!), Helaine Alessio and Kathleen Marron (get in shape for your ears and your life), and Mark Ross (a personal idol of mine; acknowledge your hearing loss, be assertive in dealing with it and use good communication strategies).

Hearing loss can be difficult and frustrating. It affects one of the most important aspects of our lives—interpersonal communication. The most rewarding thing about my career was being able to help people hear better and deal more effectively with their hearing loss. Reading this book will help anyone with a hearing loss become better informed and hopefully inspire them to take positive actions to improve their lives.

At this point, you might be thinking, "So what's the bottom line Dr. Hawkins? Are you going to walk on to the bridge to healing and start the journey to better hearing after reading this book?" I will give you all the details in the Foreword to the next edition.

David B. Hawkins, PhD
Professor Emeritus
Mayo Clinic, Florida

CHAPTER ONE
Aging and Hearing Loss
James F. Maurer, PhD

Dr. Maurer completed his studies in Audiology at the University of Oregon Medical School in 1968. In 1971, he developed and directed the first mobile auditory testing and rehabilitation program in the United States for low-income older persons, which functioned for almost two decades. His efforts in Costa Rica establishing an Audiology diagnostic testing clinic, which bears his name and his University, earned him a Governor's Commendation. He was also instrumental in the discovery of a new hereditary deafness syndrome. He has written and co-authored nine books and many articles on hearing loss and aging. After heading the Audiology program at Portland State University for twenty-five years, Dr. Maurer retired as a Professor Emeritus. This chapter is in memoriam and remains timeless.

This chapter remains dedicated to those of you who are 50 years and older. It's also written for your friends and relatives who wish to understand the causes and consequences of hearing problems as they relate to aging. In reading these pages you will discover strategies for helping the person with hearing difficulties.

More than 34 million Americans are affected by hearing loss and fully two-thirds are over the age of 55. Among the chronic health conditions of the 65 and older group, hearing impairment ranks near the top. Also, almost half of this population has at least two chronic health conditions, and this trend appears on the increase. Over age seventy the incidence of hearing disabilities increases to nearly 50 percent. Unfortunately, loss of hearing is more prevalent than ever in history, yet the gradual course of auditory aging is not the primary cause of this problem. What has changed since the 1960s is the increasing acceptance of noise—a topic we will re-visit.

Hearing instruments have continued to advance technologically. The most revolutionary advancement is probably the "Open Fit" (also called open ear or open canal) hearing instruments that are largely invisible to the observer and can be fit to people with mild through moderately severe hearing losses. But this new design is especially friendly to seniors with characteristic audiograms that fall off in the high frequencies and physical handling difficulties experienced with some other types of hearing instruments.

Many older persons listen to music, although a hearing difficulty may interfere with their enjoyment. Since a typical hearing loss during the aging years robs them of higher pitch sounds that are audible to normal hearing people, the hearing-impaired tend to increase the volume in order to make the music more audible, sometimes to the discomfort of others. A problem with this adjustment is that when the music is made louder, lower pitch notes become amplified as well, and may register as being too loud for some listeners like the guy beating on the wall. Emphasizing just the high notes can be helped somewhat by changing the tone control to high tone emphasis, if such an adjustment is available on the television set, radio or stereo system. Of course the hearing sense is much finer tuned than the tone control circuit in a stereo. The enhancement of higher frequency notes is better accomplished with a properly fit and appropriately tuned digital hearing instrument.

Another factor that interferes with listening enjoyment is a phenomenon called "recruitment." Recruitment is the abnormal growth of loudness that may occur among some persons with sensory hearing losses. These individuals react aversively to loud sounds, such as shouting, banging on metal, sharp high-pitch sounds and even loud music. They require special care in the selection of appropriate hearing aid characteristics.

It's important to know that when you take charge of any sensory limitation with proper eyeglasses, hearing instruments, etc., you're really taking care of your brain, the single most important organ in your body. When your ears transmit sounds to the brain as electrical impulses, it's the brain that actually hears. And when your hearing aid helps you hear high frequency sounds in music or in speech, these "new" sounds reach the brain and it immediately "plasticizes" the experience.

In its healthy state the brain is plastic, busying itself with establishing neural networks that represent your new activities. Ageing behaviors, such as continually seeking comfort, being reluctant to try new activities, ignoring the changes going on around you, and adhering to the "old ways" of doing things fail to release the neurotransmitters that signal plasticity. You've given up and so has your brain. You're on a downhill slope with no skis. In other words, your aging behaviors foster more aging.

Some good advice to counter these problems is published by The Dana Alliance in conjunction with AARP and its educator community, National Retired Teacher's Association (NRTA).[1] Based on recent brain research, the manual advises the following to forestall mental decline:

1. <u>Use your Mind</u>: Challenge yourself intellectually by reading, discussing, stay socially connected, challenge yourself.
2. <u>Exercise</u>: Engage in frequent aerobic exercise, push yourself.
3. <u>Make a Difference</u>: Feel in control and believe that what you do makes a difference on a day to day basis.
4. <u>Stay in School</u>: How long you stayed in school is linked to life-long brain health. Continue learning.
5. <u>Don't Do Drugs</u>: Excessive alcohol (more than three drinks a day) and illicit drug use are hazardous to brain cells.
6. <u>Protect Your Head</u>: Using seat belts and helmets greatly reduce the risk of sustaining head or spinal cord injury.
7. <u>Manage Stress</u>: Chronic stress is known to damage nerve cells. Decreasing stress improves memory performance.
8. <u>Be Heart Healthy</u>: Even in the early stages, diabetes or atherosclerosis (fat hardened in the arteries) increases the risk of cognitive decline. Both conditions may be preventable and both can be treated medically.

Which brings us to memory: An older couple came into my office for a second opinion. Urged by her husband, the woman had purchased two hearing aids, that she was wearing with some discomfort. Upon examining her I found that her hearing was normal for her age. In this instance, the husband's perception of his wife's "hearing impairment" was incorrect.

Additional testing revealed a problem with short-term memory. Her husband would ask her to bring something from another room, and she would interrupt her activities in the kitchen to do what he asked. Then when she got there, she forgot what it was that he wanted. He took this to mean that she didn't hear him, which was not so. She had simply forgotten. All of us forget at any age, but forgetfulness happened often with this woman.

As we get older, it takes us longer to store new information, especially when our mind is on something else. We hopefully don't have Alzheimer's disease, although memory loss is one of the first signs. But if memory difficulties impair day-to-day functioning and are of concern to others, seek a qualified specialist, usually a Doctor of Psychology or Psychiatry. There are psychological tests and other forms of evaluation, such as imaging and disease markers in the blood that can provide a diagnosis. But don't wait. You're most likely to discover that like most of us your memory difficulties may have increased with aging.

Did you know that a loss of hearing might reduce your memory ability? The research going on by Dr. Arthur Wingfield and his colleagues indicates older folks with hearing loss take longer to process spoken messages. Part of the reason for this is that they expend time and energy trying to understand what is being said. Researchers believe that this effort may also impair their memory. They tested older adults with mild to moderate hearing losses and found that so much cognitive energy was spent on trying to hear accurately that they forgot what the message was all about. Even when aging persons can hear the words well enough to repeat them, their ability to remember these words was poorer in comparison to older persons with good hearing.

According to Dr. Wingfield: This extra effort of straining to hear during the initial stages of speech perception uses up processing resources that would otherwise be available for transferring the spoken words into our memory. Wingfield called his study a wake-up call to anyone who works with older people, including healthcare professionals, to be especially sensitive to whether hearing loss may interfere with memory function. He suggested that those who talk to older persons should speak clearly and pause between "chunks" of meaning without dramatically slowing down the speed of talking. The objective is to provide the hard of hearing person with clearer speech and greater time to understand and remember.

Psychologists have known for years that aging affects our ability to recall things in the immediate past more so than our ability to remember the distant past with our "crystallized" intelligence. Does this mean we get dumber as we age? No. Does it mean we aging persons have trouble with a task that requires *new* learning? No, but our minds may not be as nimble as they used to be. Does it mean we're more likely to forget someone's name after just being introduced than a playmate's name recalled from childhood? Yes! Is this a new problem for us? No. We've forgotten things stored in short-term memory all our lives because we were distracted or focused on something close.

We can compensate for our memory decline by gaining more knowledge on a daily basis. This wisdom that we accumulate builds more neural networks in our brain, irrespective of our age. If our attitude is positive and we engage in daily activities, we are unconsciously keeping our brain healthy and open for more learning.

Thus neural pathways are established to represent the effort of our new experiences. Stroke patients who have lost the use of a limb can be helped, not by learning to use the good leg to compensate for the deficit, but by repeatedly focusing on movement of the paralyzed limb. The brain responds to the forced movement of the "dead" limb. Neural connections are formed that fuel hope for success in giving life to the damaged muscles. Similarly, allowing a hearing aid to recover lost sounds that have long been missing in your listening experiences creates positive, youthful changes in the brain. Even in the later years of life the brain can remain plastic, responding to new experiences and learning.

There are many older persons who can put up with a few misunderstood conversations and neither they nor their friends perceive loss of hearing sensitivity as a problem. These people are a fortunate minority. However, these same persons may have difficulty hearing when messages are spoken too rapidly or spoken in background noise or spoken in other forms of interference that limit their ability to understand. These problems are in the brain, not in the ear. The aging brain conducts messages much slower than in former years. This means that we process incoming information more slowly than a 15 year-old grandchild. Some of us can identify with these problems and the frustration that result, not from our inability to hear, but from our inability to understand messages.

Even in a fairly quiet place there's a greater problem paying attention because of auditory and visual interference. ("Great sermon wasn't it?") The drone of sounds and happenings that become neural noise may be someone coughing, or the neighbor's leaf blower, or a feather on someone's hat that keeps moving because of a breeze or whatever happens as a diversion. Even our thoughts at the moment can interfere with our ability to concentrate, causing us to make poor judgments or create a momentary lapse of memory, such as when driving a car. "Honey, you just missed our exit!" We older folks simply cannot handle as many inputs as we used to, and it's harder to focus on what we're doing when there are multiple hearing, visual, or even touch or smell challenges. I find the person using sign language during a newscast somewhat distracting, yet I know that what he's doing is invaluable to extremely hard of hearing people. Still I find myself missing information because I can't seem to avoid looking at him. His actions are interrupters—the neural noises that interfere with my hearing and understanding.

We have always believed that our brains could perform several tasks at once, like the disc jockey who listens to his headphones for a network announcement while he busies himself with a CD that he's going to air, while he is reading a commercial. It may seem like he's accomplishing three tasks all at once and therefore his brain must be capable of focusing on three different activities simultaneously. Rene Marois, a professor of Psychology at Vanderbilt University has researched the "bottleneck" that occurs in the brain: "We were interested in trying to understand limitations, and in finding where in the brain this area called *information bottleneck* might be taking place. We found that tasks as simple as pressing a button when a visual stimulus appears caused a delay in brain function." So despite common belief that the human brain is built for multitasking, this Vanderbilt scientist believes that our cerebral center is nothing more than a one-trick pony. For example, while driving a car in heavy traffic and talking or listening on a cell phone, your brain must direct your attention to only one activity. If it happens to select the cell phone activity, then your attention to driving is at risk. That certainly explains drivers who are "asleep" at the wheel after the green light flashes.

A highway accident study found that 80 percent of automobile crashes are caused by lack of attention. We older folks are more vulnerable than younger generations, whether we like to admit it or not. Our reaction time is slower, our eyes admit less light than when we were younger, and we're more than likely to have a loss of hearing however slight. Coupled with these limitations and for some folks a dozen other restrictions, we're more susceptible to interference than in our younger years.

Aging behaviors like sitting in a rocker dozing or watching TV day after day don't cause the release of neurotransmitters that signal new plasticity in the brain. Instead such behaviors increase the aging process in the brain. The same thing happens when we spend too much time thinking about or acting upon thoughts or actions that are reruns of our younger lives. The brain further deteriorates. But give the brain something new to deal with and it will return an increased level of plasticity and higher level of performance. Put a little zest in your life!

The brain is the center of our universe of communication. It is the brain that hears. It is the brain that understands. The ears merely provide the input that the brain acts upon. When a message is distorted because of a hearing loss, the brain may not be able to recover it or it may recover it incorrectly. But if a hearing instrument effectively clears up what the damaged ear is missing, then the brain acknowledges the communication and the message is understood.

As our hearing gradually diminishes during the aging years a slow adaptation takes place. We unconsciously adjust to our change in hearing sensitivity and equally unconsciously avoid places or people or activities where our difficulty is most manifested. My father, who spent his last few years at Crystal Lake in northwestern Montana, once remarked to me one evening. "You know, there aren't any crickets around here anymore. I used to listen to them at night before falling asleep. I wonder what wiped them out?" When I returned home I sent Dad a small, portable listening device and some batteries. I told him it was a "Cricket Catcher" and maybe it would help him hear a few other things too. I received his letter a few weeks later. He thanked me and sent me a list of things he could hear again, from the teakettle whistling to the little scratch that a flying squirrel makes when he lands in a nearby tree close to the deck. And of course the crickets.

Living with a Hearing Loss

Even a slight hearing impairment during this time of life may occasionally affect our ability to understand others. Since the voices of people with whom we talk vary in those characteristics that contribute to understanding, we misinterpret some individuals more than others. Voices differ in pitch, loudness, quality and output (words per minute), each of which can influence the clarity and intelligibility of the speaker's voice. Words spoken are more understandable for some voices than others. The clearer speaking person utters words that are more precisely formed, or articulated at a speed of around 250 words per minute. Tell that to your television station newscaster who's a talking marathoner.

Obviously, teenagers can keep up with the accelerated speech of their age group. But many of us cannot. We simply have to ask them to speak more slowly. Broadcaster "hype" has turned "hyper" for many of us who remember all too well the comfortably paced, resonant and clear voices of the golden age of radio and early television. Today radio and television stations that still endorse clear and reasonably paced communication are not as easy to find. Since some voices are clearer than others, it pays to shop around the networks or look to public broadcasting for better listening experiences.

Visual cues, seeing the speaker as she or he is communicating, contribute to our getting the message. But constraints in our communication environments differ considerably. Some places are worse than others, where messages spoken reverberate from bare walls and floors and are lost in the wake of their own noise. In rooms containing carpets and drapes that are farther away from outside traffic noise, interference is minimized. Something to think about if you're apartment shopping.

Places where older people congregate should be stellar listening environments. Unfortunately, this is not always the case. I recall visiting a dozen or more senior adult centers, noting the fact that while most were clean and pleasant, many were located in high noise areas and few attempts had been made to reduce interior noise. One center was actually located under a roller skating rink!

If you're reading this because you have an older parent or grandparent with hearing problems, keep in mind that it's much easier to converse with them in a quiet room. Make sure there's good lighting and try to maintain a speaking distance of less than nine feet. You'll be pleasantly surprised at how much easier conversation becomes and how much stress is reduced.

Background sounds around us can also be a positive experience. We constantly monitor the world we live in, often unconsciously. Our hearing sense, as well as our vision, keeps tabs on what is happening in our space. There's often comfort in the constant background of sounds and sights in our environment. There is a sense of belonging.

Like brush strokes on a canvas, the myriad of small sounds that we're so accustomed to hearing tell us we are a part of reality. They also contribute to our sense of security. Detection of some warning signals may be challenged by our hearing loss, sounds such as footsteps on carpet, tires on soft snow, or even fire burning in the next room. Hearing loss dampens the enjoyment of some activities that gave us pleasure in the past: theater-going, music appreciation, religious services, watching television, dining out, having a drink in places with background noise, talking to others on the telephone. Even a mild hearing loss can reduce life satisfaction for some things we once took for granted. But we must persist in these life satisfaction experiences by sitting closer to the speakers or the person speaking, or wear hearing aids or get a telephone amplifier and push ourselves to admit, "I'm a little hard of hearing. Could you speak a little slower and louder?" Again, your brain will thank you.

There is an acoustic issue that afflicts a few of us. We are all blessed with tiny tubes that extend from the back wall of the throat (behind the nose) into the middle ear cavities of each ear. The purpose of these Eustachian tubes is to ventilate the middle ears with fresh air. The tiny mouth of each tube is normally closed, but may open when we yawn, cough or snore, thus permitting air to come in. However, the mouth of the aging tube may tend to remain open in some cases. This condition is not something to get excited about, but for some persons it creates the complaint, "My voice echoes." And sometimes when they wear hearing instruments that amplify their voices, they say, "My voice echoes a bit louder." So an open Eustachian tube can cause voice echo, and wearing a hearing instrument may make this echo a little bit louder. Some people are troubled by this and some are not. Hearing care practitioners are experienced in helping those who are uncomfortable with this condition. The new "Open Fit" hearing instruments are built to reduce or eliminate this phenomenon.

None of us are alike. We differ because of genetic influences, environmental effects, and luck of the draw injuries and diseases that can damage us permanently. The specific problems that we encounter with our hearing deficit also differ, as do our physical and emotional capabilities to overcome adversity, lifestyle, support system of friends and relatives, tolerance for breakdowns in communication, the severity of our hearing impairment, and how we go about pursuing professional help. What we have in common is that we will circumvent a lot of future problems by seeking quality professional help in getting evaluated and discovering the resources available to us.

Other Influences that Affect Hearing

The amount of loss that we accrue in growing older can be compounded by the consequence of exposures to other events or agents that damage our hearing mechanisms from infancy onward. These include noise exposure, diseases, high fever, head injury, toxic chemicals and drugs, blood supply deficiency, lack of oxygen and genetic influences.

While the Occupational Safety and Health Administration (OSHA) has required noisy industries to provide ear protection since 1970, this partial solution came too late for many who are now retirement age. We live in an industrialized society where noise is seemingly omnipresent. We were endowed with eyelids to keep out most light while sleeping but no "earlids" to suppress background

9

sounds of traffic, air conditioners, hair dryers, and a host of other noise sources that are pervasive in our homes. In fact, we are indeed fortunate if we can sit in the quiet security of the living room, close our eyes, and hear nothing.

Both community and recreational noise has increased over the years with the rise in population and proliferation of noisy vehicles and gadgets. Intrusion by other peoples' noises in formerly quiet neighborhoods often taxes our patience and our hearing ability. Automobile speakers, boom boxes, iPods in the ears, chain saws, lawn-mowers, firearms, noisy vehicles and 50-plus years of Fourths of July all have a cumulative effect. (See Chapter Two, Q&A #6)

Other places include jazzercise facilities, which often feature loud music, and where the most vulnerable ears are infants parked in strollers in the same room. Beauty salons can be very noisy, but fortunately some manufacturers of hair dryers are now building quieter machines.

Older men often spend time in home workshops, where electric drills, saws, sanders and other equipment can add to the hearing loss associated with aging. The intrusion of jet sleds, all-terrain vehicles, snowmobiles, high volume music in unwelcome places, such as parks and wilderness areas add to mental confusion and the physical demise of delicate inner ear structures. Shooting high-powered rifles, magnum pistols and shotguns is a very efficient way to lose decibels of hearing as well. In fact, conventional ear protectors do not completely protect against such firearms. And usually we don't even know our loss of hearing sensitivity is happening until it's too late for it to recover.

Old age hearing loss and noise-induced hearing loss can combine to produce a greater hearing impairment. We can't turn the clock back and start wearing ear protectors at an earlier age, but there's something to be said for protecting what hearing we have left. I carry an inexpensive pair of foam earplugs for use on long airplane trips and other situations where noise exposures may be loud or lengthy. I find it interesting, having provided hearing tests on a number of rock musicians back in the early 1970s, that many who were slow in requesting help on hearing protectors now seek advice on hearing instruments. I wonder about the hearing sensitivity of their audiences, the baby boomers, who are now a part of our aging population. Our children and grandchildren seem to perpetuate the thirst for loud music, despite our warnings and presentiments.

Adjusting to Hearing Loss

Do you remember when someone younger first called you "Sir" or "Madam"? Did you experience a momentary flicker of surprise, an evaporating thought that you somehow must be different from that moment on? It was as if you had suddenly arrived on some plateau in life from which there is no return. Interestingly, our arrival may have more to do with our biological age (how old we look and feel) than our chronological age (how many birthdays we've celebrated). Some of us look our age, some of us don't. Realization of our hearing difficulties can be like that, when someone younger gives us the bad news, "Dad, you've got to do something about your hearing!" We are different from that moment on. However, for many of us there's no sudden realization. Since our loss of hearing sensitivity is usually gradual, it may take us a long time to recognize and acknowledge that we have a problem.

An older gentleman living in a townhouse called this to my attention. "We used to hear the clock ticking." He said. "I suddenly realized I don't hear it anymore."

"What concerns me," his wife added, "is that I don't hear any of the little sounds anymore. When I'm folding clothes I don't hear what I'm doing. And I used to be able to hear the gas when I turned up the stove. It's interesting that some rather important sounds in our lives disappear without a whimper."

Hearing old sounds again is like visiting old friends. It's a very positive experience. Some of us don't accept hearing loss so readily. And this lack of acceptance creates a quandary for the specialist trying to help us.

John was a 70 year-old longshoreman who came to my office announcing that his physician told him he had the arteries of a 30 year-old. He flexed his triceps and asked me to feel them. "Hard as steel," I responded, knowing what was coming next.

"Doc," he shouted, "I don't have any trouble hearing. I don't know why they sent me here. I can hear a pin drop."

But he couldn't. In fact, he couldn't hear a brick drop. Not only that, he couldn't understand conversational level speech. And ability to hear in noise? Forget it!

I always have great compassion for such patients. I know they want to stay young. They want to have youthful hearing skills. They don't want to wear hearing instruments because they see them as another indication that their bodies are growing older. But not tending to the needs of our ears is like letting a garden go to weeds. And that garden is our brain.

Another reason why denial takes place is manifested in the slope of the hearing loss associated with aging. We hear low pitch sounds a lot better than sounds that are high pitch. For example, we can hear the sound of a soda can dropped on an enamel table, but we can't hear the fizzing sound of the escaping soda. Thus, telling this person, "You're not hearing!" is not entirely true. Some sounds, the low ones, may be heard quite well. Others, the high ones, may not be heard at all. Nevertheless, our ever-active brain tries to fill in the blanks, sometimes correctly, sometimes not.

Grandpa and his grandson Joey were painting the shed. Joey said, "Gramps, let's go get some **thinner**."

Grandpa laughed and shook his head incredulously. "**Dinner**? Why son, we just had lunch!"

This illustrates the difference between <u>hearing</u> and <u>understanding</u>. Joey's grandfather *thought* he heard the message. In fact, he correctly heard five out of six words spoken by his grandson. But he didn't hear one critical consonant—the soft, high pitch /*th*/ sound in the word "thinner," so his brain tried to fill in the blank with "dinner." This small misperception changed the entire meaning of his grandson's request. When this starts happening to us frequently in conversations with others, it's time to ring the bell for help!

The high frequency loss may create a quandary for us when we *see* a bird singing, but don't *hear* its song, or when we only see the whisper of wind in the trees. Missing some sounds also can be an unnecessary annoyance.

A gentleman in his fifties told me, "I couldn't understand why every time we went to the cabin I ended up with more mosquito bites than the rest of the family. Then one time my daughter pointed out that there was one buzzing around my ear. I realized suddenly that I hadn't heard it!"

A few indomitable individuals take immediate and aggressive action to counteract a recently discovered hearing difficulty. One elderly gentleman bounced into our hearing center like a bandy rooster one morning, gesturing wildly and shouting, "How do I get some hearing devices?" When I asked him why he thought he needed them, he said that he no longer could understand his patent attorneys at board meetings. "I have to depend on what they say. Trouble is they mumble separately. If they all mumbled together," he quipped, "I think I'd understand what they were talking about. I invented a new type of truck hoist and I want to get it patented."

He wanted a quick solution, and he wasn't about to let a hearing impairment stand in his way. This was a man who was used to making adjustments. He was 82 years old. Did I say "old?" I mean *young!*

Often our reluctance to seek help presents a barrier to those attempting to talk with us. If straining to hear is fatiguing, imagine what it must be like for another person who has to keep repeating all day. The denial of aging is often projected as a stigma against hearing instruments that are for "older" persons. This can become an attitudinal disclaimer that hearing difficulty is not an important part of our lives. A glass of water won't suffice when we're thirsting for the Fountain of Youth. Some of us even engineer our lives to convince ourselves that we hear normally. We simply minimize our exposure to situations where the hearing deficit compromises our enjoyment of life!

I asked a woman in her late fifties, "What things did you do ten years ago that gave you a lot of satisfaction? " She responded, "Let's see, I was very active in the church. I really enjoyed that. I taught Sunday school. I went to a symphony about once a month. Oh, and bridge club. That meant a lot to me ten years ago."

"Are you still enjoying these activities?"

She was quiet for a moment. Then she blinked a tear away. "Well no, not really," she shrugged. "It became too much work teaching those children, and too much fussing to get ready for the symphony. I moved onto other things, I guess."

As we talked on, it became clear that she had sacrificed part of her life satisfaction because of increasing hearing difficulties. She had carefully limited her activities so that the impairment wouldn't affect her life. And she had accomplished this without ever admitting that the cause of her withdrawal was her inability to hear. Fortunately, this woman turned out to be an excellent candidate for aural rehabilitation group counseling. Once she could identify with other women in the group who had similar problems, her self-esteem increased and she began to move out of her self-imposed isolation.

What's also missing here is social responsibility. We hard of hearing people owe others the right to conversations that are free of frustration. We owe our friends freedom from continually having to repeat conversations. We owe them an honest appraisal of our hearing difficulties. What is not realized by many of us is that once we can hear better, we may discover a rebirth of more youthful participation in social activities. We become better social companions. As one wife exclaimed, "When he puts those digital instruments on, he's more like himself!"

Retiring Comfortably with a Hearing Loss

It's interesting to talk to people with auditory problems who have recently retired. Some experience a sudden loss of power, the ingratiating experience of sliding backwards down the slope that leads to non-person status in the eyes of once admiring co-workers. Normal hearing people may experience the same thing. This was the feeling that a recently retired physician related to me. His repeated returns to his beloved medical school, where he had held an office for more than thirty years, were met with disengaging smiles and chafing comments like, "What are you doing back here?"

He began questioning whether a prejudice was occurring because of his whiter-than-others' hair, the fact that he was retired or perhaps his new hearing instruments. Ultimately, he felt that his once respected opinion no longer mattered, and with some reluctance, he ended his visits.

Some years later after my own retirement, he called me. "You know," he said, "if you ever write another book or have to counsel a lonely retiree, you might remember this piece of advice: if you live alone and your world is passing you by, be grateful for what you have left. Then make yourself important to someone. You'll be pleasantly surprised how important you become to yourself." He was embarking on his third trip to China to help children with birth defects. He had decided that nothing could get in the way of his need to help others, neither hearing aids, aging body, nor unresponsive colleagues.

We are a diverse population, we older persons. Some of us cross over to retirement more slowly, tenaciously clinging to our previous roles in life through occasional work or social and service activities. We may express joy at having left our working selves behind. We network with friends seeking a newfound freedom, finding companionship in the excitement of long-awaited travel, new recreational activities, educational pursuits, or greater involvement in hobbies. Some of us don't retire at all.

Hearing loss does not respect our differences. We find individuals with auditory difficulties in all lifestyles. What's important is not to let this problem curtail our pleasures in life. A pharmacist friend who had been a trap shooter since boyhood was left with a significant high frequency hearing impairment in both ears. He wears two hearing instruments in retirement, and when I visit his home I always take a handful of earplugs. He constructed a woodworking shop in his garage and now creates quality furniture both as a hobby and to supplement his pension.

Regaining life satisfaction may mean letting go of some of our former attitudes about aging and hearing loss, and beginning to accept the realities of a new emerging self. It helps to take stock of all the positive attributes in our lives. There are people who like us for who we are—wrinkles and all. They could care less about our need for prosthetic devices. They care about us. They accept our baggage. In fact, it becomes so much a part of us that the people we care about don't even see it anymore.

It also helps to look around at the place where we spend most of our waking hours. What are the positive attributes in our home environment? What things produce pleasure for us? If we close our eyes, how many of these things would no longer be pleasurable, such as a picture that is dear to us or a good book? If you could close your ears and hear nothing, what things of enjoyment would be missed? Take inventory of positive activities outside the home, things we like to do with our time. This could include hobbies, meetings, entertainment, and activities that are more physical, such as walking, fishing, travel, golf. If we apply the same limitations to our activities, in turn, closing our eyes and ears, what would the effect be? What enjoyable activities would we have to give up? What we discover from this simple exercise is that first, there are many positive things operating in each of our lives. Getting older is not a virus that takes away all our satisfaction with life. Second, recounting our pleasures with one of our senses "closed" eliminates many positive aspects of our lives that we would not give up willingly.

Now hang onto that thought, because not giving up is exactly the attitude that must persist if we are to realize our most positive potential in spite of our hearing loss. This means accepting ourselves wearing devices that will open up a part of the world's pleasures that would otherwise be forsaken. It means accepting our new selves.

Interestingly, the world will accommodate our new self-image, and we can now move forward with our lives. People began to like us better because we are *real* in projecting who we are, and we're happier for that experience. Popeye probably said it best, "I am what

I am, and that's what I am!" Did he wear hearing aids? You mean you didn't notice?

During the aging process, we consciously or unconsciously make other adjustments as well. Knowledge of reduced physical stability makes us move more cautiously in risky situations where we might fall, such as walking down steps, getting into the bathtub, climbing a ladder. We discover that sudden movements can produce dizziness or unsteadiness, so we avoid quick changes in position. Diets may change to cope with various health conditions after age fifty. We find ourselves getting less sleep at night because of wakening, and may discover a decrease in the quality of sleep. So we may compensate with naps. And the list goes on.

Compensating for perceived changes is a healthy, friendly way of insuring survival and happiness. It's taking charge of one's life. It's making a positive statement about the aging years! Like the old adage that a graying dowager told me years ago, "There may be snow on the roof, but there's fire in the furnace!" And stoking that furnace, managing one's life experiences, reducing the impact of a hearing difficulty by acknowledging the problem to others, getting professional help, and arranging living places so you can hear better, are giant steps in the right direction.

Helping Yourself

Arranging where we reside, eat, work, play or pray means getting closer to the source of sound, i.e., TV set, stereo, religious pews, or the waitress in a café. What we're accomplishing by favorably positioning ourselves in living situations is improvement in understanding communication. The greater the distance we are from the sound source, the more distortion we'll experience, whether we realize it or not. Besides, there are those visual cues: facial expressions, mouth movements, gestures, and body language. These nuances of visual communication may not be visible from a distance, but do help to actually clarify the message up close.

Stage-managing our lives also means getting away from distracting or overpowering noise or loud music. One may enjoy the power of organ music and sit close to it in a place of worship, but at what cost to hearing the message? If one ear is better than the other, favor the "good" ear. Think of places in your life where it's difficult to hear: sitting in the back seat of an automobile, sitting in a breakfast nook adjacent to the humming of appliances, standing at the cash register in a busy restaurant, or before the agent in a bus terminal. Make a list of these noisy places in your life and then think of alternatives.

Helping a Loved One in a Restricted Environment

If you know someone in a nursing home is benefiting from hearing instruments, keep tabs on their ability to use them. Does this person have the skills and dexterity to put the instruments in the ear, turn them up, and remove them before going to bed? Can the individual change the batteries when appropriate? Is the family physician checking to see that the ear canals are free of wax buildup? Can someone on the nursing staff peek in the ear with a pen light? Are there complaints of hearing aid whistling? This "feedback" can be caused by earwax. Is someone remembering to open up the battery doors at night, saving on battery life during sleeping hours and allowing air to circulate through the hearing instruments?

And while we're at it, is anybody cleaning this person's glasses once in a while? Remember, visual skills also help the hard of hearing person. If your loved one can no longer manage prosthetic devices, ask who in the nursing staff is responsible. In many cases I've witnessed, the primary person who cares and oversees the maintenance of your loved one's prosthetic devices is you!

Strange things happen to hearing aids in nursing homes. They can be stolen, substituted for someone else's instrument down the hall, uncomfortably stuck in the wrong ear, chewed on or digested by someone's visiting dog or cat, dropped in the toilet, plugged with wax, sentenced to lifetime solitary confinement in a dresser drawer, stepped on by a 250 pound attendant, or awaiting invitation under the bed to the fraternal order of dust bunnies.

If the instrument seems to be helping the older person only by making him or her more alert, take this as a positive sign and reward the use of hearing aids. If you make a visit and find it's not being worn, check to make sure the aids are working. It's wise of you to participate in getting the hearing aids in the ears during your visit. Chances are your warm gestures of touching, smiling, talking and caring will have positive consequences on this special person. And on you as well.

You may be reading this book to find out what you can do for a loved one who sadly can no longer understand the printed word, cannot write effectively, or may be wandering in that personal void associated with significant cognitive decline. Unfortunately, the lower the level of intellectual functioning, the poorer the prognosis for gaining much benefit from amplification. But check first to see if increasing the volume of the soothing sound of your voice seems to create a pleasant experience, or even an increase in understanding.

I took some graduate students to a nursing home to do hearing testing on some residents. One gentleman sat very quietly in a corner of the hallway not socializing with anyone. He just looked emptily at the opposite wall. One of the staff told us he had been diagnosed as having Alzheimer's disease. We had brought with us a powerful body hearing aid with a big red volume control. We placed it in a harness on his body, hooked his right ear up to it, and slowly began turning up the volume. His mouth opened slightly, his head turned toward us, and as we watched, a wisp of a grin turned into a full-fledged smile. One student tried to subdue her excitement and quietly asked, "Can you hear me?"

He looked at her, lips moving, eyes glistening, and managed an, "Uhhh" and shook his head "Yes!" A few weeks later, after we had showed him how to use the aid and charge the battery each night, I returned to see how he was doing. I found him sitting on the sun porch, holding hands with an elderly woman. The big box with the red volume control hung like an Olympic medallion on his chest.

References

1. Dana Alliance for Brain Initiatives. *Staying Sharp*: NY, 2006, p. 3-4.

CHAPTER TWO
The Emotions of Losing Hearing and a Bridge To Healing

Richard E. Carmen, AuD

Dr. Carmen received his Doctor of Audiology Degree from the Arizona School of Health Sciences, a division of the Kirksville College of Osteopathic Medicine. His professional interests have encompassed human studies research, clinical practice and hearing aid dispensing. He has authored and co-authored a number of books, chapters, and more than 50 papers—most peer-reviewed. In addition to writing extensively in the field as a regular contributor to various professional journals and publications, his interest in patient education and consumer awareness has led to a number of articles published in nationally recognized periodicals. He currently resides in Sedona, Arizona.

One benefit of ever-expanding technologies in the U.S. includes improvements in hearing aid designs and circuitry. In essence, hearing aids are getting smarter and "prettier." They've become less obtrusive and offer superior performance than just a few years ago. With the advent of telecommunication devices such as Bluetooth cell phone systems, wearing anything in the ear these days is at best passé, and perhaps even fashionable. For some, I've noticed that it seems to have become a statement of moving with social change. Have you noticed how comfortably people now talk into thin air using Bluetooth devices stuck in their ear? Thus, there really should be minimal cosmetic concern today over visibility of anything in the ear. It's hard to tell the difference between telecommunication devices and some state-of-the-art ear-level hearing aids. Some hearing aids are so elegantly designed that they no longer even look like hearing aids, perhaps more closely resembling fashion jewelry— they even come in pink!

This has culminated in profound social change, a shift in thinking by both wearers and observers whereby the stigma of wearing these devices that don't look like hearing aids is essentially gone. When we authors were completing the first edition of this book in 1997, such a thing was only imagined. However, while we've transformed negative judgments in only a matter of a few years through more appealing designs, there remain other issues to address.

Your first reaction to learning you have hearing loss and must wear hearing aids can still hit some people like a brick. By the time a practitioner determines you have hearing loss, you've already been living with it most likely for years, so you're just getting confirmation of what you already suspected. Even so, for many it's a hard pill to swallow. For some, it rattles them to the core. As Quasimodo, the Hunchback of Notre Dame said in his dying breath as he lay in the arms of the beautiful gypsy girl La Esmeralda, a tear rolling off his cheek, "Why could I not have been made of stone?" His torment reflects that of many of us—the pain of *feeling*.

However, *feel* we must, as this is what characterizes us as human. Emotional experiences may be wonderful, painful or sometimes perplexing. Yet, more than our physical body, feelings are the substance of our identity. Each of us reacts differently toward the varied experiences of our lives. For centuries, fields of study have been devoted to exploring this fascinating phenomenon, but the search seems to have yielded as much controversy as knowledge. From more than three decades of clinical practice, I've observed some compelling emotions and feelings in my patients. These observations have extended into my own family members with loss of hearing, so the feelings we'll be talking about touch home—deeply.

I once taught an audiology course to graduate students where I had them wear earplugs for a day, morning to bedtime. They were asked to log their feelings and emotions and report to the class the following week. We were all overwhelmed by two things: the similarity of their experiences and the depth of their emotions. Students reported they felt inadequate and incompetent. There was also a sense of limitation in areas they had taken for granted. Simple tasks like using the telephone couldn't be performed without special manipulation, difficulty or strain. Common sounds like ice stirred in a glass, running water or turning a page in a book—sounds that orient us in our environment—were gone.

Driving the car was a new experience. With the absence of wind and traffic sounds, there was a feeling of disorientation. Students quickly realized how important their vision became to compensate for what they could not hear. And yet such compensation felt inadequate. By the end of the day most of the students confessed they were worn out and disturbed by what they had gone through.

"What a horrible experience!" one student remarked.

An apt description I thought.

One student reported she had collapsed into bed crying. Others were unnerved or dispirited. Their collective reactions were directly linked to feelings of inadequacy, a deficiency in their daily performance relative to what they expected or how they were accustomed to functioning. Once the earplugs were removed, all ill feelings dissipated. Their sense of normalcy and calm returned. If your significant other has no idea what it feels like to have a hearing loss, this would be an enlightening experience.

While this experiment was useful to normal hearing students, it revealed what you no doubt already know. Hearing is an essential human sense. Its absence would be greatly missed by anyone. As hearing declines, similar to other sensory deficits, we humans have an extraordinary ability to compensate for the loss. Such compensation is a built-in defense mechanism to which we give little thought. It just happens. If you have a heart attack, the body works quickly to establish other pathways and connections. If you lose your sense of smell, your eyes become more probing. When vision diminishes, listening can sharpen. And when hearing declines, you might overcompensate in other ways, also by listening more attentively. Your innate ability to exclude extraneous sounds might kick in. You might cup your hand around your ear. You may find yourself focusing sharply on the person speaking, unconsciously observing lip, facial and body movements and gestures. This very natural tendency happens without much conscious awareness. And these things do help you "hear" better. In fact, they work so well that the very act of compensation can fool you into believing that you hear okay. It's for this reason that loss of hearing might have given you the impression of being so insidious.

"It just kind of crept up on me!" you might have thought. Of course it didn't really.

Something you've probably said many times in your life, and will see repeated, rephrased and reanalyzed in this book is the complaint, "I hear, but I don't understand the words clearly!" This is particularly true when trying to communicate in a group, around a few people or in an environment with background noise such as in a restaurant or automobile. Early on, when you had problems hearing, you may have passed it off as being no more troublesome for you than for anyone else in the same situation. But as issues around poor hearing grew more apparent and the process of communication began breaking down, you must have realized the problem was not going away.

People who develop hearing loss from an explosion, accident, physical trauma or rapidly progressing disease are probably more inclined to deal with it because it's so sudden and unmistakably apparent. But if you're in generally good health and are the type of person who doesn't like to think of yourself as less capable than anyone else, you might have found that you started blaming other people for frequent miscommunication. This is very common. You may think others are not speaking clearly or loudly enough, or they "mumble" their words. It's only when sufficient numbers of people close to you suggest that it's you and not them, that you might have gotten your first inkling of something within your personal communication system has gone awry. Some people never come to this realization and go on believing that others are the source of their communication failure. They continue to blame other people and are discouraged that others appear to enunciate so poorly. Nothing will deteriorate a relationship faster than denial. This is not healthy in any family, and why it's so important to establish the core issues.

Our ego is quite attached to our overall health. Most of us like to think of ourselves as being in shape with a good heart, strong bones, good vision and acute hearing. For some of us, admission of poor hearing is like admitting we've given in to old age. It's like a forced resignation we never invited. The realization of hearing loss places you at a crossroads, offering two quite opposing paths. The first is to admit the hearing loss; the second is to deny or ignore it. The former decision (admitting it) allows you to reassess and seek solutions to enhance and maximize your quality of life. The latter decision (denial) negatively impacts every aspect of your life, and can destroy relationships and decreases your quality of life.

To resist the reality of having hearing loss perpetuates miscommunication and the turmoil that goes with it. If we try to ignore loss of hearing or stop thinking about it, the problem persists. For some people, the crossroads for acknowledging hearing difficulty, but doing nothing about it is where they get stuck for years. In fact, the statistical odds are very high that prior to reading this book you've known of your hearing loss for more than five years, during which time frustration, communication problems and hearing difficulties have significantly increased.

Problem-Solving Ground Rules

Before we discuss your feelings about hearing loss, let's first define the terms used and establish the ground rules upon which problems can be solved. "Hearing loss" is the physical condition in your ear. "Hearing difficulties" pertain to specific situations (like struggling to hear someone speaking to you). A "hearing problem" is your internalization of the situation, how you process the issues surrounding these situations (like getting upset at your spouse or yourself if you miss a word).

These terms are often mistakenly interchanged. If you're in the living room watching television with your family and you realize you're missing too much dialogue, you might ask others in the room if you can turn the volume louder, in which case you think you've solved the hearing difficulty. The reality is your family will object to having the television too loud. This may make you annoyed or you may feel rejected, angry, resentful or other ill feelings—a sure sign of a hearing problem. You're internalizing feelings about a hearing difficulty. As stated earlier, the first step in solving difficulties about your experience is to first acknowledge the challenge, then recognize how you feel about it. A willingness to consider your hearing loss as a fact of life will create a solid bridge to healing. This is the foundation upon which all hearing problems can find resolution.

There are two common philosophies people seem to adopt once hearing loss becomes part of their lives: cover up the fact that they have it or tell others when the occasion is appropriate that you don't hear well. There are many variations between both themes, but if you look at yourself honestly, you'll recognize your own pattern.

The emotions a person feels when hearing loss is confirmed incorporates the full range of human experiences. Some are relieved that at last they know that this is the cause of their problem, that they're not losing their mind, and are grateful at the diagnosis. At the other extreme, some are horrified. It seems an unbelievable possibility that the problem could be wholly theirs. "Surely most people mumble!" they conclude.

So many of us react in so many different ways that predicting how you might experience hearing loss is quite a complex matter. Furthermore, your reactions to hearing loss do not necessarily correlate to the degree of impairment; that is, you can have a mild loss of hearing which impacts your life more profoundly than someone with more significant hearing loss. Your reactions will be most influenced by how you feel about yourself and the world around you, your personality type, and how other people close to you deal with your problem. The most important ground rule to bear in mind when looking at your issues as we progress through this chapter is, *you must be honest with yourself.*

Self-Inquiry

If you're willing to be introspective about your hearing problem and consider solutions, this is the place to begin. Problems usually have at least two solutions that bring about healing: (1) change the situation, or (2) change how you feel, interact or react. The problem with *changing the situation* (if you're an unaided person with hearing loss) is that you could find yourself continually changing your environment and still not hearing well. You may also try to change the environment to avoid an unpleasant experience, but it doesn't necessarily help you hear better.

On the other hand, the problem with *changing how you feel* is that it's an imposing challenge. It's very difficult to transform anger into love, frustration into understanding, or embarrassment into delight. Surely, it would seem that it doesn't happen quickly if at all. Nonetheless, it can happen. When people open themselves up to accepting hearing loss, change can occur very quickly. It's the most predictable criterion on which hearing aids will be found acceptable; perhaps even the only criterion. Changing how you feel about hearing loss and hearing aids also becomes apparent to others in your life, and by your acceptance, relationships transform.

The definition of "change" is "giving up something for something else." The difficulty for anyone in making changes is that it requires giving up something to which they've grown accustomed. It feels less certain and sometimes frighteningly unfamiliar. Most of us find we're not skilled in making changes. It's usually something we find uncomfortable. Even good changes are known to cause stress. A move to a better house, getting a higher paying job or even winning the lottery cause high stress. We tend to want to stick to "the familiar." Yet, going from dysfunction to adjustment necessitates change. To avoid stress, most of us unknowingly tend to stick to bad situations. I've often thought that there should be a course teaching students during their last year of high school how to effectively make changes in their lives. How better adjusted to life we'd all be.

Perception has everything to do with the degree of adjustment, acceptance and solutions you embrace with regard to your hearing loss. Many people with hearing loss report they have altered their view of the world around them in an unhealthy way. People who were once soft spoken and gentle sometimes have become outspoken and annoyed; others who were once alive with spirit and energy may have grown pensive and withdrawn. Those close to them notice these changes and are saddened by it. If you aren't aware of such changes, if in fact they exist, it could be because they usually develop slowly over a period of years.

If you have the courage to really look at the impact hearing loss has had in your life, the following exercise may prove to be revealing. When completed, read the same list to someone who knows you well (your spouse, a grown child or a close friend) and ask this person to respond *how he or she believes you operate in the world.*

Exercise #1

If the statements feel mostly accurate, write True; if they feel mostly inaccurate, write False:

1)_____I don't hear well because other people mumble, don't enunciate clearly enough or talk too softly for me to hear.

2)_____Since I've had this hearing loss, I can't do all the things I'd like to do.

3)_____People don't dare make jokes about my hearing trouble in my presence.

4)_____I don't mingle with as many people (old and/or new acquaintances) as I used to because I don't hear well.

5)_____I just can't be seen wearing a hearing aid.

6)_____If I'm left alone in a conversation, I don't understand or trust what I hear.

7)_____I know people think I'm not as sharp as I used to be because I don't hear as well as I once did.

8)_____If I don't want to hear what someone says the first time, I'll remain quiet; it's a waste of my time trying to hear when I can't.

9)_____I just can't seem to assert myself the way I used to (or as others do) since I lost my ability to hear well.

10)_____It's difficult for me to accept I actually have a hearing loss.

11)_____I know I'm the source of the problem because of my hearing loss; when I miss what somebody says, it's not their fault.

12)_____Even though I have a hearing loss, I still do all the things I used to do.

13)_____I have humorous things happen to me as a result of my not hearing well.

14)_____In spite of my hearing loss, I'm careful not to give up any relationships I have in my life, or lose out on any potential relationships, by staying home too much.

15)____I would not think of hiding the fact that I was wearing a hearing aid.

16)____I feel completely at ease communicating with anyone in most environments even though I have hearing loss.

17)____Despite my hearing loss, other people do not think less of me than before my loss developed.

18)____I don't mind asking people to repeat what was said if I didn't hear it.

19)____As my hearing loss has developed, I have made a systematic effort to compensate for it by being more outgoing.

20)____It's easy for me to think of myself as having a hearing loss.

Note: Before you read the following interpretation which will give away the design of this exercise, be sure you and your partner complete it fully.

Interpretation

Statements 1 through 10 are the reverse of 11 through 20, respectively. For example, statement 3 is opposite to statement 13. There are two built-in veracity checks: one is that however you responded to a particular statement, if you're honest with yourself, you should have responded opposite to its corresponding statement. The other check is the way in which your partner responded.

Did you respond consistently to both sides of the statements, True on one, False on the other? Did your partner agree with you? If not, you may want to look carefully at the content of those statements. Are you procrastinating? Do you spend a lot of time with negative thinking about your hearing loss? Are you blaming others?

Or is your outlook healthy? Do you tend to think more positively in handling your hearing loss? Do you try to find the lighter side? Are you just as engaged in life as before you developed loss of hearing?

Once you've examined the way you and your partner responded to the same statements, you may well find that you are the one person who has prevented finding your own solutions. This exercise was not an attempt to change who you are, but rather, to *change and improve how you interact in the world.*

Denying Hearing Loss

If your hearing healthcare provider informs you that you have an irreversible sensorineural hearing loss, despite the fact that today more than 35 million other Americans share the same challenge, this is not necessarily the news you want to hear. However, it's quite another story if you don't believe it or choose to do nothing about it.

Most standard dictionaries define *denial* as *the refusal to believe* or *the act of disowning*. It's rejection of the notion that your hearing is an issue. In so doing, you not only disown the condition, you decline help because logic dictates that you cannot seek help for something that does not exist. Although true denial of hearing loss is rare, resistance to help is common. The following kinds of refrains are ones you yourself may have made:

- "I just ask people to speak up!"
- "Nobody hears everything!"
- "It doesn't bother me!"
- "Don't talk to me from another room and I hear great!"
- "Only my spouse complains about it!"
- "I ignore it!"

Often, early resistance provides a useful function by allowing people time to recover from the initial shock of knowing they have a hearing loss. But some trap themselves here for years. To resist the notion of hearing loss implies you hear well, and this resistance is really self-deception.

Mechanisms of resistance can become an integral part of the way people operate in the world. The more sophisticated and highly developed their compensatory responses, the easier it may be to deny the problem. For example, some may have others help them hear, like asking others to repeat, rephrase, speak up and so forth. Without realizing it, they may grow skilled at favoring an ear, tuning one person in and another out, repeating what they think they hear to confirm its accuracy, reducing background noises, making educated guesses, watching facial movements and expressions as well as gestures and body language. These are all excellent cues and necessary ways to hear and understand better, but as suggested earlier, the irony is people can get stuck believing all of this will solve their problem. It doesn't.

If you're wondering if you're experiencing resistance to hearing loss as you read this book, go back to the previous exercise to know. If you were in true denial, you probably wouldn't have picked up this book in the first place (although you could read it and say, "That's not me they're talking about!"). If you're well aware of your own hearing loss, but deny its presence when others inquire, that's not denial, it's concealment. So, congratulations! At least you're willing to look at the problem. This is where we must begin.

It's been said that uncorrected hearing loss is more noticeable than hearing aids because the act of concealing a hearing loss is doomed to fail. It can make a person appear foolish, inattentive, disinterested, confused, senile or cognitively impaired. A person operating at this level needs to understand the serious emotional hardships imposed on oneself, the spouse, family and friends. Denying, resisting or minimizing the impact the loss has in one's life (or in the life of others) does not solve the problem. Having others "hear" for you is not the answer either. In fact, these things compound the problem in close relationships. "Why should I carry the burden?" an honest but resentful spouse will ask!

You might feel annoyed that you have a hearing loss, but your spouse is annoyed that you do nothing about it. You may isolate yourself from family gatherings because you can't hear, feel foolish or embarrassed, but your family feels abandoned and dismissed that they aren't important enough to you if you isolate yourself. If you're a person unwilling to seek help, it can even create the feeling in loved ones and friends that you're selfish or irresponsible.

Co-Dependent Behavior

I published the results of a study in 2005[1] that explored who audiologists felt were more resistant to hearing aids, men or women? Over half of the practitioners surveyed (about 54 percent) reported they felt men were more resistant; about 34 percent felt it was equal; and only 9 percent of respondents reported women as being more resistant. If you're a man resisting the notion of hearing aids, so long as family members continue to serve your endless listening and hearing needs by repeating what you miss, interpreting messages, allowing you to avoid the telephone, without the need for you to seek professional help to solve this problem, you're in a co-dependent relationship.[2] In fact, your spouse may have become so good at this behavior that it fools you into believing you actually hear adequately! That is, she has essentially become your ears. In some relationships this may be cut short once the hearing loss progresses. In other relationships as hearing loss gets worse, the spouse is Johnny-on-the-Spot and feels an increased demand on her to help you, digging an ever deeper trench into co-dependence. Either way, it's co-dependence and it's not healthy. More than anything, it deprives you of your <u>hearing independence</u> which translates to social isolation, the very thing we need to prevent as we get older because aging alone can cause isolation. To compound it by untreated hearing loss would be a shame.

In my patients willing to give up co-dependency, I've seen a rebirth of marriages, newfound love and warmth among family members (especially children so frustrated and angry at the unwillingness to get help), and even greater work efficiency. Regarding the latter, I have put hearing aids on a few psychiatrists in my career who had finally reached the end, unable to hear their patients correctly. Hearing aids change lives.

Isolation

The personal tragedy of untreated hearing loss is the isolation that results from avoiding all the situations that make hearing a challenge. These also happen to be the situations that have made life so enjoyable. These include avoiding plays, movies, maybe giving up a favorite restaurant because it's too noisy, even giving up a certain relationship or two because someone speaks too softly.

Ultimately what this can lead to is the sense that you live in your own world. Once you've broken away from the "outside world," your reality is made up of two rather distinct and separate worlds: yours and the outside world. The longer you remain separate from this outside world, the more alienated you can feel about it, the more fear you can develop about having to deal with it simply because it's no longer comfortable and it's no longer safe. The natural progression of this can be giving up more and more pleasures in life in order to operate more efficiently in your ever-shrinking social world. The healthy resolve is to face the need to address this self-imposed "exile" from these pleasures by seeing if hearing aids are the answer. This is an enormous bridge to cross for many people, but it can be the bridge to healing.

Procrastination

Making the decision to try hearing aids is not an easy one for some people, especially if sometimes you hear beautifully, and other times poorly. Loved ones may also observe this to be true. This gives the false impression that you have a *listening issue*, not a *hearing problem*. This is the elusive nature of hearing loss because it's frequency-sensitive. That is, you may hear your father perfectly, but cannot hear a co-worker. You may believe room acoustics are the problem or that it's other people—they talk like they have marbles in their mouth or "mumble." You may hear people differently because some voices project better than others. Men are usually easier to hear than women or children for those with high frequency hearing loss. And the environment plays a significant role, especially in noise. The configuration of loss you have may allow you to hear some voices well, others poorly. (See Chapter Eight)

Putting off the hearing evaluation (or hearing aids) can be based on what seems solid logic:

- "I'm too young!"
- "It's not bad enough yet!"
- "No one I know likes their hearing aids!"
- "We just can't afford it now!"
- "After we paint the house!"
- "Tom has a hearing loss and doesn't wear hearing aids and he gets along just fine!" (but of course Tom really doesn't).

Such people recognize their hearing loss but try to find every excuse not to do anything about it. This is procrastination. Hearing problems may be minimized in order to justify not pursuing treatment. And in the presence of other health concerns, this may seem like just one more issue on the list:

- "After I do my teeth!"
- "I don't want to spend my children's inheritance!"
- "If only Medicare paid for it!"
- "Maybe after that trip to Hawaii" (or that new car)

Any of this sound familiar? If so, we'll explore this more thoroughly. Now fasten your seatbelt!

Emotions Behind Hearing Loss

How you deal with hearing loss probably parallels how you deal with life. We all develop patterns by three to five years of age which become programmed into who we are. While you may wish to act and react differently, to a certain extent, it means deprogramming (and reprogramming) yourself. Despite such imposing challenges against change, to attempt change precludes the *desire* or *intent* to change. As you are about to discover, failure to change by not seeking help for your hearing loss is linked to a myriad of emotional issues, some permanent, but most preventable.

I encourage anyone willing to explore their internal emotional processes to consider consulting a psychotherapist (individually or as a couple). Such an unbiased personal sounding board so often proves to be a very rewarding, productive and nurturing experience.

Let's explore some of the emotions we commonly see in people with untreated hearing loss.

Avoidance, Anxiety & Social Phobias

As presented earlier, aging often correlates to isolation because with progressing years we lose friends and relatives, it becomes more difficult to get out, we have less energy, and so forth. Thus, we can find ourselves isolated. Untreated hearing loss compounds the matter. The experience of separation from others is not limited to the over-fifty crowd. I've seen many patients in their twenties and thirties give up their favorite activities because of their inability to hear adequately. I've seen high school students refuse to wear hearing aids because they feared peer ridicule. They sadly preferred to be left alone and miss out on social interaction rather than risk being seen wearing hearing aids. [Howver, since the advent of open ear hearing aids in 2003, this situation has improved.]

Social phobias can and do commonly develop from untreated hearing loss.[3] A social phobia is a form of anxiety; a persistent fear of social or performance situations in which embarrassment may occur. For example, if you avoided a particular social obligation with your significant other because you feared the embarrassing consequences of your hearing loss, and these situations were persistent, excessive and recurrent for more than six months, you probably have a social phobia.

If you've noticed that you've been avoiding social situations as described, you should be concerned. Fundamentally, you're cutting yourself off from the nurturing people who make you feel loved. Clearly not a healthy choice. Apart from hearing loss, anxiety disorders are serious medical conditions affecting more than 40 million American adults and can grow progressively worse if untreated.[4] Through the 1990s, anxiety disorders in the U.S. grew by more than 50 percent and posed a major public health concern. Interestingly, according to the National Academy on an Aging Society (http://www.agingsociety.org/agingsociety/pdf/chronic.pdf), hearing loss is the third most prevalent chronic condition in older American men. So, if you're an older American gentleman experiencing hearing loss, you have much greater risk for isolation and avoidance of common pleasures in life—not to mention depression.

Depression

More than 26 percent of Americans ages 18 and older suffer from a diagnosable mental disorder in a given year,[4] and major depressive disorder is the leading cause of disability in the U.S. for ages 15-44.[5] Onset of depression usually occurs in the twenties, impacting twice as many women as men. Unfortunately, for those with hearing loss, the likelihood of also suffering from depression is increased.[6]

Although these are staggering statistics, it's important to understand that depression is not a natural part of aging. It can be prevented and is treatable in about 80 percent of older adults. A major source of depression, especially in older adults, stems from untreated hearing loss. The simple action of wearing hearing aids can resolve the associated depression. In older adults, this should be pursued aggressively, since depression is also commonly associated with anxiety and other ailments. As we age, our normal coping abilities diminish. It's so important to restore as much normal functioning as we can, at any age, but especially in these later years.

Often we think that what we feel inside remains hidden. It is easy to forget that those we love can usually see past this thin veil. And rest assured, if depression is there, and they love you, they'll eventually see it, and will be suffering along with you. In clinical terms, depression is often described as *anger turned inward*.

Anger

Anger is a kind of stepchild to depression. When left untreated, people with depression can be difficult to be around, but something you may be surprised to hear is that you have a right to be angry! It's your body. Hearing is a needed and vital sense. Its loss influences almost every aspect of socialization. Every time you ask people to repeat themselves, it's a quiet reminder of a problem that does not go away. A natural response can be anger.

The problem with anger is that it typically finds its outward vent. Eventually, some can become resentful and angry at others over their own need to have things repeated. Worse yet, they may become angry when a family member suggests they should get help! They already know that. They just don't want to hear it from anyone. For some, this is just too painful.

The dynamics of this emotion are fairly simple. A person becomes angry that they're not hearing. The family is upset that this "stubborn person" isn't doing more about the hearing loss. Some hard of hearing people, oblivious to the impact their hearing loss has on others, may ask to have things repeated in a blaming manner. This leads others to feel that the communication problem extends to them, and therefore their anger gets them angry!

If you recognize that anger is an issue, you may also discover that you're as angry (or disappointed) with the world as you are with yourself. This further locks you into the separation crisis between "your world" and the "outside world" mentioned earlier. Perhaps you desperately want to make a change and escape from your world, but don't know how or where to turn. Seeking audiologic counsel is a first step. Indecision may keep you angry and upset. If you continue ignoring the problem, the issues surrounding it are further perpetuated. If you find solace in reverting to denial of the problem, it's a short-lived reprieve because you've already awakened to the truth of your situation.

For many people, unexpressed inner turmoil finally shifts from its simmering hidden view to boiling over. People around you are less likely to understand from where this hostility arises, especially if you yourself are not in touch with it. You risk relationships with friends and family disintegrating as fast as your quality of life.

If you're of an angry nature and if it's hearing loss-related, hopefully you will become attuned to the fact that your upset originates from your failure to seek help. Thus, no one but you can really solve this dilemma. Through such awareness, you'll also discover a renewed sense of calm because now you can take back control of your life.

Selfishness and Resentment

If we ever question how difficult it is to live with another person, all we have to do is look at the divorce rate. Health issues aside, it's not easy. Now throw into the mix a partner who refuses to get help for a health problem, regardless of the condition. Now you have a problem. If this problem is untreated hearing loss, a common reaction of a partner is anger or disappointment that their loved one will do nothing about the problem. This then, in very subtle ways, begins to characterize you as a person.

Coming to terms with hearing loss can be a very slow journey for many. If you expect others to compensate for your loss of hearing instead of assuming this responsibility yourself, as mentioned, you'll likely set up a fertile environment for strained family relationships. Your negligence may rightfully be seen as a selfish act. Of course you're entitled to expect others not to speak to you from another room or in the presence of such cacophony as a loud television, a vacuum cleaner or music. But in the absence of wearing hearing aids, the family shouldn't be expected to manipulate the household for your convenience, especially when it's at the expense of others you care about.

If you're out socially without hearing aids, you already know how frustrated your friends and loved ones are over seeing you miss out on conversation. If you're in a movie theater (if in fact you're not avoiding theaters altogether) and your spouse or friend must continuously repeat the onscreen dialogue, you might be hearing a lot of, "Shhh!" from those seated near you. In the meantime, you, your partner and maybe others around you have just missed another line of on-screen dialogue.

Eventually, for most every relationship, all the rigmarole required by loved ones to accommodate your hearing problem at the expense of their untold inconveniences will lead to resentment. Why has your problem suddenly become their problem? Why is it their responsibility to be your ears? Why should they be solving your hearing problems?

Frustration and Defeat

I've already presented frustration as a common experience surrounding untreated hearing loss. When you look at such family dynamics, frustration touches about everyone. It's very easy for family members to forget that you do not hear well. After all, there's no melon-size growth on the top of your head to remind them, no bandages, no walker. Because you give the general appearance of looking so normal, others may expect you to *hear normally*. Your kids or spouse may continue to talk to you from other rooms, or with a back turned or with a pencil in the mouth. Inadvertently, your loved ones are aiding and abetting without realizing it.

Worse, you tell your physician that you believe you have some hearing loss and are surprised what you're told. Research has shown that, first, your physician will not test you nor will he or she likely refer you to a hearing healthcare professional. To add insult to injury, you could be told: "Don't worry about it. Everyone gets a little hearing loss eventually. I have some myself, but I just ignore it!" If you're told to ignore it, this may be well-intended advice, but it's misguided and will likely add to your mounting frustrations. Know that you are not alone. Only about 86% of U.S. physicians screen for hearing loss.[7] This suggests that if you're to get help, you must be the motivator.

During the initial stages of hearing loss you may have actually laughed at many misunderstood words. I was with my wife at the hardware store when I thought she said, "Do you need some *coffee?*"

I took the comment personally because I incorrectly assumed she thought I was not paying attention, but she had said, "Do you need some *caulking!*"

One time when we were about to get dressed for a party, I asked my wife what I should wear. She turned to me and as clear as a bell said, "Leave your clothes!" Leave my clothes? Hardly, I thought! I only heard it correctly when she repeated it. "*Leisure* clothes!" Good thing she repeated it!

I've also experienced hearing everything seemingly quite clearly, but none of it making sense. And I have normal hearing! Repeating doesn't help because with a hearing loss at specific frequencies, the same words are expressed at the same frequencies where you don't hear well. Therefore, it's more important to have someone <u>rephrase</u>.

The humor of mistakes seems to eventually dwindle. What remains are the day-to-day frustrations. This can culminate into mixed emotions as we've discussed, especially annoyance and anger fueled by frustrations. A frequently heard comment by the person with hearing loss, as well as the family is, "I can't stand it anymore!" In fact, the longer untreated hearing loss persists, the greater the frustrations <u>for everyone</u>.

When frustration upon frustration over years occurs, there's a real sense of defeat by everyone in the family, including you. You may make every effort to hear. You may listen, struggle, are attentive and make every effort to connect to this outside world, but it entails so much frustration and defeat that it can become easier to withdraw. In almost every other health problem, you'd have received treatment. You wouldn't have put yourself and your loved ones through these hoops. To do nothing is resignation, concession, submission and surrender. It does nothing to lessen the burden on others. Such inaction is actually self-defeating, and shouldn't even be an option. (If you already wear hearing aids and feel defeated, explore all other choices available to you, *many included in this book.*)

Embarrassment

Probably the single most common experience among people with untreated hearing loss (and their family) is embarrassment. Second-guessing what you think you hear, offering inappropriate responses, missing the punch line to a joke, or getting wrong directions are small examples of what you and loved ones experience. Struggling to hear can put others ill at ease.

Research indicates that some sufferers do not pursue help for themselves because the thought of wearing hearing aids is embarrassing. Ironically, failure to get help usually proves to be more embarrassing. With the open ear hearing aid fittings of recent years, this trend has shifted. The cosmetic appeal of these exceptionally inconspicuous hearing aids has attracted wearers who would never have considered amplification on any other basis. As a result, embarrassment about hearing aid use has significantly diminished, and in many cases it's even been eliminated. In the hearing health-care treatment of today, hearing aids and other appropriate amplification accessories offer anyone with loss of hearing the most efficient avenue to independent hearing. These devices allow you to break free of your dependence on others and can make all the difference in strengthening your relationship with those around you rather than fueling embarrassment and other ill feelings by ignoring the problem.

Rejection

Bill was a likeable but boisterous man. He told funny jokes, but he told them with such volume that strangers thirty feet away laughed. He was a source of constant entertainment as well as embarrassment to his wife and friends. Sitting in a restaurant he'd talk about people's personal problems. It wasn't that his friends didn't want their problems discussed, they just didn't want the entire restaurant to hear about it. It was as if Bill had no sense of where he was or what was appropriate. No one suspected, until I met Bill, his wife and others for lunch and recognized a marked loss of hearing. Bill knew it, but he wasn't about to let anyone else in on his secret. His refusal for help cost him the relationships of people who once truly loved and cared for him. However, his friends simply could no longer tolerate the humiliations that went along with the friendship.

Many hard of hearing people are rejected by others who do not recognize their condition. When others remain uninformed about why you may behave or interact the way you do, they're forced to draw wrong conclusions that carry undesirable consequences. You don't have to be vulnerable to social rejection. You have to experience this only a few times to know how painful it is. People may whisper behind your back, "Is he senile?" "Is he functioning okay?" "Does Bill know he constantly offers incorrect replies in conversation?"

The ultimate rejection is you rejecting the outside world, continuing to live isolated in your safe but narrow space of not hearing well.

Sensory Deprivation

Sensory deprivation research was popular in the 1950s and told us much about the human experience in the absence of stimulation. John Lilly, MD[8] authored a few pop culture books on this subject matter, as well as fascinating scientific papers. He was the creator of the "Lilly Tank," where you could float on Epson salts sealed inside a tank, had no body awareness, no light and no sound.

As auditory, visual and sensual input diminishes with less stimulation to corresponding neural centers in the brain, the brain is not happy. Lilly's students subjected to these experiments generally could not tolerate the absence of sensory stimulation longer than a few hours or a few days. Besides altered realities, other complaints included feelings of disorientation and inability to concentrate. You should know that people who suffer from hearing loss (which is auditory deprivation) also report *the same symptoms*.

Solitary confinement in prisons is a recognized method of sensory deprivation. Over time, it has been shown to cause permanent problems, most profoundly, *intolerance to social interaction*. Obviously, this effect is counterproductive to a society that desires paroled inmates to be acclimated back into society. By no coincidence, symptoms found among many people with untreated hearing loss (auditory deprivation) also include *intolerance to social interaction*. This is the "My world / their world" scenario.

Much of reality (what little we understand of it) is based on our very delicate sensory systems. Impairment to any one of our five senses *does result in an altered state of reality.* If you miss portions of communication and don't realize it, you're experiencing one thing while something else entirely may have been intended. When you experience auditory deprivation, your natural instinct is to avoid social situations because just like students in Lilly's experiments, not many people like living in an altered state of reality.

There's now reliable scientific evidence to document the fact that untreated hearing loss can lead to a variety of unhealthy emotional conditions. The Hearing Instrument Association in conjunction with the National Council on Aging ran a study with over 2,000 hard of hearing adults and over 1700 family members.[9] This study concluded that people who suffer from hearing loss were more likely to experience increased anger, frustration, paranoia, insecurity, instability, nervousness, tension, anxiety, irritability, discontentment, depression, being temperamental, fearful, more likely to be self-critical, suffer from a sense of inferiority, social phobias, be perceived as confused, disoriented or unable to concentrate. Experiencing only one of these would seem enough to inspire one to seek help, but unfortunately, many people with hearing loss tend to experience a variety of these unhealthy emotional states.

Furthermore, research shows that failure to stimulate hearing (the auditory portion of the brain) by not wearing hearing aids may result in a more rapid decline in speech recognition[10-11] and brain atrophy.[12] These reports were based on a substantial number of subjects who possessed at least a moderate degree of hearing loss in both ears, but received only one hearing aid. As a result of auditory deprivation in the unaided ear, a reduction in speech recognition occurred. For some, when hearing loss is not addressed as a major health issue, the risks of negative emotional impact are high. These are consequences that can be avoided, but often are not because people don't realize the impact of untreated hearing loss. Now let's examine this impact.

Your Spouse or Significant Other

Probably the average person with hearing loss has experienced impatience at times causing them to be harsher on loved ones than they'd like, or insensitive, unkind or unfair. Once you've recognized your actions, you may feel guilty. You may wish you could have handled the situation differently, but you just couldn't control yourself. More so, you may feel like it's a vicious cycle—you expect loved ones to be your ears, yet, those around you get fed up doing the hearing for you. It seems to be lose-lose.

In my consultations I always included the spouse because they are the richest source of information. When I ask for their assessment, the common response is, "I'm so tired of repeating myself!"

What you must understand is that everyone feels the same way. Even if you live a substantially isolated life, your hearing problems are woven into the lives of those who hear, especially at home.

Sadly, only 20 percent of people who suffer from hearing loss seek treatment through hearing aids. This speaks volumes about what spouses endure. It does not only mean louder television, repeating yourself throughout the day, and filling in parts of important conversations, it dangerously raises the level of anxiety in a healthy spouse married to someone with hearing loss. Your spouse may develop her or his own anxiety around your issues, which can start with annoyance and lead to anger, intolerance, a sense of hopelessness, and can even lead to depression. In some cases, I've seen my patients divorce. Struggling to communicate under these circumstances is exhausting.

Many people with untreated hearing loss feel they're not ready for hearing aids. Inspiring you to seek this needed help may be the most challenging task your spouse and family face. Change of course begins with your readiness. The rewards can dramatically improve lives and usually transforms relationships.

Expectations versus Actual Performance

If you're a person living in a non-amplified world, you no doubt have expectations about hearing that may not align with your performance. I've had my own family members with hearing loss refuse hearing aids, then go into situations expecting to hear. At the end of the evening, I'd point out how much conversation was missed.

People who haven't yet come to terms with their loss of hearing, or who have not fully admitted it to themselves, mistakenly believe that *they hear all they need to hear.* The truth is, *you only hear what your hearing capacity permits.* The illusion to oneself is two-fold: you not only fail to get important information, but you don't even know it. The illusion to others is they think communication has occurred when in fact it hasn't. Thus, we not only have miscommunication, but multiple altered states of reality.

Exercise #2

Here's a little exercise that can help you better understand hearing loss. Divide the top of a blank sheet of paper into three sections: on the left, title it "Situations;" in the middle "Expectations;" and on the right, "Actual Performance."

List three to five situations or environments where you expect to hear regardless of whether or not you actually can. Your task is to rate the items under the "Expectations" and "Actual Performance" columns by selecting one of the following ratings:

NEVER - RARELY - SOMETIMES - OFTEN - ALWAYS

After you've completed this, take another piece of paper and list the same situations. Then have your partner or someone close to you complete how they think your expectations versus actual performance pan out. This makes for healthy discussion and a great opportunity to compare and contrast perceptions. The more truthful you are with yourself, the more you'll gain from these insights.

Interpretation

If you rated everything in the exercise the same for all situations, either you're an amazingly well adjusted person with hearing loss or you're kidding yourself. It's unlikely that all hearing situations on your list will be evaluated equally even if you're well adjusted.

So, take a closer look at your list. Bear in mind that people with normal hearing will rate the situations of expectations and performance differently because of their varying listening environments. The difference indicates the magnitude of the problem; the greater the difference, the greater the problem. For many people with loss of hearing, it's typical to have expectations higher than performance levels. As a result, reactions to environmental situations that prove difficult can lead to the emotions we've discussed.

Moving into Acceptance

Are you ready to make a positive change in your life? Do you want better communication? Do you want to do more to help yourself? Is the quality of your life important enough to you to make positive changes? Do you care enough about loved ones to make these changes? Can you accept that the "outside world" is safe enough for you to coexist?

You already recognize the trials and tribulations of inadequate hearing. By now, I'm sure you could write a book about it! Acceptance of hearing loss allows you to move on. It's that easy. You know that despite all your efforts, all your loved ones' efforts to compensate for you not hearing, nothing has probably worked. This realization is essential before you can move on with clear vision. Coming to terms with the emotions surrounding your hearing loss not only builds that bridge to *hearing*, but a bridge to *healing*. Acceptance of your hearing loss allows you safe passage into the outside world.

References

1. Carmen R. (2005) Who are more resistant to hearing aid purchases—women or men? *Audiology Today*, 17 (2).
2. Carmen R. (2005) How Hearing Loss Impacts Relationships: Motivating Your Loved One. Sedona, AZ: Auricle Ink Publishers.
3. Carmen R and Uram S. (2002) Hearing loss and anxiety in adults. *The Hearing Journal*, 55 (4).
4. Kessler RC, Chiu WT, Demler O & Walters EE. (June 2005) Prevalence, severity, and comorbidity of twelve-month DSM-IV disorders in the National Comorbidity Survey Replication (NCS-R). *Archives of General Psychiatry*, 62 (6): 617-27.
5. The World Health Organization. (2004 update) The global burden of disease. Table A2: Burden of disease in DALYs by cause, sex and income group in WHO regions, estimates for 2004. Geneva, Switzerland: WHO, 2008.
6. Bridges JA & Bentler RA. (1998) Relating hearing aid use to well-being among older adults. *The Hearing Journal*, 51(7): 39-44.
7. Kochkin, S. (Oct 2009) MarkeTrak VII: 25-Year Trends in the Hearing Health Market, *The Hearing Review* 16 (11): 12-31.
8. Lilly J. (1972) The Center of the Cyclone: An Autobiography of Inner Space. New York: Bantam Books.
9. Kochkin S & Rogin CM. (2000) Quantifying the obvious: the impact of hearing instruments on quality of life. *The Hearing Review*, 7 (1).
10. Silman S, et al. (1984) Late on-set auditory deprivation: effects of monaural versus binaural hearing aids. *Journal of the Acoustical Society of America*, 76: 1357-62.
11. Silman S, et al. (1992) Adult-onset auditory deprivation. *Journal of the American Academy of Audiology*, 3: 390-96.
12. Peelle JE, Troiani V, Grossman M, et al. (2011) Hearing loss in older adults affects neural systems supporting speech comprehension. *Journal of Neuroscience*, 31 (35): 12638-43.

CHAPTER THREE
What the Experts Say:
Your Questions and Answers
From the Editor

As in the previous three editions, this section covers questions and answers not addressed elsewhere in this book. We strive to address the most important issues pertaining to your hearing loss and better hearing, so the questions developed here are ones you yourself might ask. As a result, the most seasoned and tenured professionals were invited to answer them. Each edition has held new questions with equally new insights from three new contributors. Dr. Lin addresses issues of hearing loss and cognition; Dr. Peelle talks about how the brain adapts to hearing loss; and Dr. Fligor offers his perspective on recreational noise. Here's what the experts say!

1. What is the effect of hearing loss on cognition and dementia?

Frank R. Lin, MD, PhD is Assistant Professor, Division of Otology, Neurotology and Skull Base Surgery, Assistant Professor, Departments of Epidemiology and Mental Health, Bloomberg School of Public Health, Assistant Professor, Division of Geriatric Medicine, Department of Medicine, Core Faculty Member, Johns Hopkins Center on Aging and Health. Among a number of investigation interests, he has pioneered research into the relationship between hearing loss and cognition.

From an epidemiologic perspective we're seeing across several large datasets that hearing loss appears to be independently associated with the risk of cognitive decline and the risk of developing dementia. By "independent" I mean studies where we have accounted for and adjusted for the effects of age, sex, race, health variables, smoking, hypertension—factors that could serve as a common cause and account for just a simple correlation between hearing loss and dementia.

We've hypothesized that there may be several mechanistic pathways through which hearing loss could directly contribute to faster rates of cognitive decline or dementia. The first idea is fairly intuitive—namely, that hearing loss can contribute to a loss of social engagement and lead to social isolation. Going back several decades, we have long known that social isolation and loneliness are direct risk factors that can contribute to faster rates of cognitive decline or dementia, and there are direct neurobiologic pathways through which loneliness leads to adverse effects on brain health through cortisol and other inflammatory pathways.

A second idea is also fairly intuitive in that hearing loss can lead to cognitive load. What this means is that if you constantly cannot hear well and your brain is receiving a degraded auditory message, the brain likely has to dedicate increasing resources to help with auditory processing. This reallocation of brain resources may then come at the expense of thinking and memory abilities. The implications of this are something that we frequently observe in people with hearing loss where a patient with hearing loss goes out with their friends to a busy restaurant, and by the time they get home they're exhausted from having to constantly strain to hear.

In brain imaging studies, we're beginning to also see direct evidence for this effect where individuals with hearing loss compared to those with normal hearing have to recruit other brain regions to help with hearing and auditory processing. A third idea for how hearing loss could lead to faster cognitive decline follows along these same lines. In neuroimaging studies now, we're observing that hearing loss is associated with structural changes in the brain, and these changes in parts of the brain important for cognition and language processing could precipitate faster rates of cognitive decline.

The critical question going forward is figuring out whether comprehensive hearing loss treatment using current best practice methods and technologies could potentially reduce the risk of cognitive decline and dementia. At the present time, we still have no idea of whether hearing loss treatment could make a difference or not. In our previous epidemiologic studies, self-reported hearing aid use has generally been associated with a weak, non-significant attenuation of the risk in cognitive decline and dementia, but these results are hard to interpret. For example, individuals choosing to purchase hearing aids are likely to be more health conscious and more socially integrated than individuals not choosing to use hearing aids. We are currently in the process of setting up a definitive clinical trial to investigate whether hearing loss treatment could reduce the risk of cognitive decline and dementia. Results from this study won't be available for at last 5 years, but in the meantime, there's no reason not to pursue hearing loss treatment.

The most important thing to keep in mind, though, is that when working with an audiologist, the goal of treatment is *not* to just fit you for a hearing aid, but to ensure that you are able to communicate effectively in all settings. This requires an audiologist who can provide the proper counseling and rehabilitation and who will discuss other adjunctive assistive listening devices (remote microphones, telecoil/loop systems, etc.) that are needed to make hearing loss treatment successful.

2. How does hearing loss affect brain activity during speech comprehension?

Jonathan Peelle, PhD is a neuroscientist and Assistant Professor of Otolaryngology at Washington University in St. Louis. Dr. Peelle's research focuses on the interaction of sensory and cognitive factors in speech comprehension using a combination of behavioral and brain imaging methods. He is particularly interested in how the neural processing of speech is affected by age and hearing impairment. More information on his research can be found on his lab website: peellelab.org.

To understand what someone says, we need to quickly and efficiently make sense of a very rapid stream of acoustic information. Although our ears are responsible for initially capturing sound, it's our brains that ultimately do the lion's share of work making sense of what we are listening to. In many ways, our brains are where actual "hearing" takes place.

This doesn't happen magically, but requires the support of mental processes including attention, memory, decision-making, and so on. These are often referred to generally as "cognitive processes" or "cognitive processing". Cognitive processing is closely linked to brain activity, because it is the biological machinery of the brain that actually performs these operations. Different networks in the brain are specialized for different tasks, and so patterns of brain activity differ depending on what specific cognitive processes are being used.

Our brains have quite a bit of work to do even when speech is presented in ideal listening conditions (that is, pronounced clearly and with no background noise to a listener with good hearing). Consider that the very first time you meet someone, never having heard them speak before, you're still able to understand what they're saying. Although the physical properties of their speech are new to you, your brain is able to map these sounds onto what you know about language, and you're able to decode these sounds into words, quite often without any apparent effort.

But what does the brain do when speech is not heard clearly?

Frequently, we are still able to extract the correct meaning, but our brains have had to work harder to do so. Interestingly, we're often quite aware of this effort (picture yourself straining to hear what a friend is saying at a busy restaurant or coffee shop). The internal experience of having to work harder during a conversation has led researchers to speak about "effortful listening." This is a general term that can be applied to both people with good hearing, listening to noisy or degraded speech, or to people with hearing loss listening to clear speech. In both cases, the brain is receiving an impoverished acoustic signal, and thus needs to work harder.

Exactly what the brain is doing to make sense of degraded speech is a matter of active research. However, there are at least two possibilities that seem likely. The first is that the brain uses short-term memory to hold onto what has been heard while its meaning is being worked out. Although this typically happens without our knowledge, from time to time we may have the experience of not understanding what someone says, only to realize a few seconds later that all of a sudden we *do* understand. This is only possible if our brain has been able to keep working on what it has heard.

The second thing our brain does when speech is unclear is to make more use of the surrounding context: It uses what it knows about words that are likely to occur near other words to decide what we've heard. For example, if you heard the sentence "Jamie likes to exercise and enjoys riding his _____," you might reasonably assume that the last word was "bicycle" or "bike," even if you didn't hear it clearly. However, this isn't a complete certainty, as other words could also fit the sentence ("horse," "tricycle," "skateboard," "dolphin")—they're just less common and therefore less likely. Making increased use of context is generally helpful, but it can also mean that less typical words are more difficult to understand.

Much of what we know about *how* our brains process unclear speech comes from functional brain imaging studies of people with good hearing listening to speech that has been degraded in some way. In a typical functional magnetic resonance imaging (fMRI) study, subjects are positioned in the scanner and listen to a series of sentences, some of which are clear and some of which are degraded. We can then look to see where levels of brain activity are different between the two types of sentences, giving us an idea of the brain regions involved in effortful listening. A consistent finding is that, indeed, extra brain activity is required to understand degraded speech. This is often localized to regions of the frontal lobe involved in speech and language processing, as well attention, monitoring and control.

A clear consequence of this extra effort is that if more cognitive processing is required to make sense of what we hear, less is available for other things we might want to do (such as remembering it). In the laboratory it can easily be shown that even when we can repeat back words with total accuracy, our memory for degraded speech is worse than our memory for clear speech. Even more interestingly, our memory for clear speech occurring just *after* degraded speech suffers as well. This happens because the increased cognitive processing associated with the degraded speech continues for up to one or two seconds after the word ends, and thus interferes with the processing of subsequent words.

Thus, when speech isn't clear, our brains need to work harder. This is true for people with all levels of hearing, although it presents a special challenge for people with hearing loss because even more time is spent in repair mode. The extra cognitive processing required to understand speech interferes with other tasks, including our memory for what we have heard. The flip side of these findings is that anything we can do to aid the processing of speech—whether using hearing aids, using visual cues, and so on—should reduce the challenge of listening, and free up cognitive resources.

The brain networks that help us communicate with each other are dynamic, and adjust to both our hearing ability and the particular listening environment in which we find ourselves. This means that we can actively participate in improving our brain's performance, which is really quite a remarkable thought indeed.

3. Many people complain about poor "speech intelligibility." Can you tell us what may lay behind this complaint for some, is there clinical assessment for it, and what are the implications for hearing aid use?

James W. Hall, III, PhD is Clinical Professor and Associate Chair in the Department of Communicative Disorders at the University of Florida in. His research interests include auditory neurophysiology, auditory processing disorders, tinnitus (and hyperacusis). Among more than 150 publications, Dr. Hall is author of *Audiologists' Desk References* and four other books.

This is perhaps best answered by providing some background. As a result of advances in auditory neuroscience, the study of how hearing regions of the brain actually function, as you've read earlier in this book, there's growing awareness that "we hear with our brain, not with our ears." The practical implication of this statement is clear—hearing assessment of children and adults is not complete until speech perception is evaluated under difficult, yet commonly encountered listening conditions. The ability to hear very faint simple sounds, evaluated with the traditional pure tone audiogram, is an example of a very basic auditory process. The simple hearing test, however, doesn't provide adequate information about real-world hearing difficulties. Some people with considerable hearing loss, as described by the audiogram, seem to do very well in most listening situations. On the other hand, if the brain is not processing sound well, then even a person with normal hearing sensitivity for faint sounds may experience serious problems with speech perception and understanding, especially in adverse listening environments. A deficit in hearing in a person with a normal audiogram is referred to as a "central auditory processing disorder" (APD). The diagnosis of APD can be made in persons of all ages. This review focuses on APD with adults.

There are different types of hearing problems that a person with APD might experience. Auditory processes important in communication that are evaluated in a complete diagnostic assessment for APD might include:

- *Auditory Discrimination:* The ability to detect small and rather subtle differences between sounds, such as two speech sounds (e.g., speech versus peach);
- *Auditory Pattern Recognition:* The ability to recognize the correct order or sequence of sounds that are strung together;
- *Temporal Auditory Processing:* The ability to quickly and accurately process what's heard, including very brief transitions between speech sounds within words and fast conversational speech;
- *Auditory Performance with Degraded Acoustic Signals:* The ability to understand speech even when some of the sounds are not clearly heard;
- *Auditory Performance in Competing Acoustic Signals:* The ability to hear well when there is background noise.

An APD may occur in a person who also has a hearing problem due to damage or dysfunction at the level of the ear, that is, a typical "peripheral hearing loss." The person with both a peripheral (ear) and central (brain) hearing loss may have difficulty hearing certain sounds, particularly when the sounds are faint, and then greater difficulty processing and making sense of the sounds that are heard. In addition, it's now well known that a variety of listener (and non-auditory) factors may influence auditory processing, among them cognitive factors (e.g., intelligence level, memory, and processing speed), attention, motivation, and language experience and abilities devoted entirely to cognition in audiology. In certain populations of patients, such as young children or older adults, these factors can play an important role in auditory processing abilities. For example, for an elderly person who has memory deficits and an overall reduction in the ability to process information quickly and accurately, the impact of a co-existing auditory processing disorder may result in a major communication problem. At this juncture, it's important to point out that APD, if not diagnosed and properly managed, often leads to a variety of psychosocial problems, including irritability, frustration, anger, loneliness, and even depression.

Auditory processing disorder is regularly encountered clinically in adult patient populations by audiologists who include proper screening or diagnostic measures in the test battery. Which patients are at risk for APD and should be considered for thorough diagnostic audiologic assessment? The increased likelihood of deficits in auditory processing in aging adults has long been appreciated for over 30 years. Up to 25 percent of adults over the age of 65 years have clear evidence of APD upon diagnostic auditory assessment. At the very least, additional audiologic assessment with sensitive measures of auditory processing are indicated when patients express concerns about their hearing despite normal hearing sensitivity, when the patient's hearing complaints are greater than those expected for the pure tone audiogram, when benefit from amplification (hearing aids) is less than anticipated, and when clinical observations and/or case history suggest the possibility of central nervous system disease or dysfunction, e.g., dementia, other cognitive deficits, stroke, head injury, etc. There is growing concern about APD in a substantial proportion of military personnel and veterans who are survivors of explosions and other combat injuries.

In short, any patient with hearing or listening complaints should be considered at risk for APD until proven otherwise. Understandably, modern day audiologists who are under growing pressure to see more patients in less time, and with diminishing reimbursement, are tempted to reject such advice as not clinically feasible. However, as audiologists we alone among educational and healthcare professionals are responsible for assessment of hearing and management of hearing problems. We haven't evaluated hearing until we've described auditory performance at the highest levels of the nervous system, and we can't expect patient satisfaction or good management outcomes if we haven't identified and addressed all of the patient's auditory complaints.

Identification and diagnosis of APD is, of course, a fruitless exercise if the information does not contribute to management and, ultimately, improved communication outcome. Decisions on which strategies are required for effective management of APD are largely dependent on an accurate and complete assessment and diagnosis. APD test findings most assuredly will affect patient and family counseling. Take, for example, an elderly woman brought to the clinic for a hearing assessment by a caring son or daughter who is very concerned about mother's hearing difficulty, particularly in noisy settings. The audiogram shows a very mild high frequency sensory hearing loss, actually not much considering the patient's age, and fair word recognition scores. Lacking further diagnostic test findings, the audiologist would be tempted to simply reassure patient and family that hearing is really quite good, and a hearing aid is not necessary. However, what if speech perception in background noise were assessed and showed a marked deficit in auditory performance? The audiologist would take a very different approach with patient and family counseling and instruction and the audiologist would offer additional forms of intervention, e.g., FM technology or perhaps a computer-based auditory training program. Findings of concomitant central auditory dysfunction in adults with documented sensory hearing loss prompt the audiologist to look into features of hearing aids that would not otherwise be considered or even warranted.

Finally, some patterns of findings for APD measures for adult patients, e.g., markedly asymmetric and/or abnormal performance, suggest the need for medical referral and diagnostic work-up for neurological disorders. Many other examples could be cited to illustrate the impact of comprehensive diagnostic assessment of APD in adult patients on management strategies and overall outcome.

4. We know that the heart carries nutrition throughout the body, including the ear. Without absorption of nutrients critical to hearing, its function would stop. For example, many people who have gone on a starvation diet as a political protest have lost some of their hearing. Since we've become so vitamin and mineral conscious, is there anything you might recommend which has been shown to positively impact the hearing mechanism?

Martin Dayton, MD, DO is Past-President of the International and American Association of Clinical Nutritionists, and is currently the medical director at Dayton Medical Center, in Sunny Isles Beach, Florida. He is licensed and Board Certified as an osteopathic physician and surgeon by the state of Florida. He is a past fellow of the American Academy of Family Practice and the International College of Applied Nutrition.

Unfortunately, no specific nutritional treatment is generally used or known to address hearing loss in all people. However, strategies do exist which may address the needs of the individual with impaired hearing, in accordance with the unique circumstances of the person. These circumstances are governed by the inherited and acquired strengths and weaknesses of the individual and the conditions under which the person exists.

A child may have an inherited predisposition to allergies and live in an environment where junk food is a staple. This child may be prone to develop a form of "stuffed ears" known as serous otitis media. Fluid accumulates in the middle ear due to allergy-mediated inflammation, swelling, and closure of the Eustachian tube. Dysfunctional pressures may develop in the ear. Infection may take hold in part due to impaired transport of immune factors to the area and impaired drainage of toxic fluids from the ear due to swelling.

On the other hand, an elderly person with an inherited predisposition to hardening of the arteries who eats the nutritionally sub-optimal standard American diet may develop progressive hearing loss. This is due to auditory nerve tissue deterioration associated with impaired circulation—accelerated with aging. Perhaps, accumulation of environmental or pharmaceutical toxic materials with time is also a role in the manifestation of hearing loss.

These two cases illustrate how diverse the contributing circumstances can be in regard to the manifestation of hearing loss. Each case must be handled differently in the use of nutrition to address the same goal of improved hearing. The child in the first example needs to avoid foods which may trigger allergies. Wheat, cow's milk, peanuts, chocolate, eggs, and soy are frequent offenders. Various methods are used to determine which foods need to be avoided, when and how often. Various methods may be used to reduce such sensitivities. Plant extracts from stinging nettles, aloe vera, citrus and seeds of grapes may reverse the allergic processes. Vitamins, such as C and pantothenic acid may also be useful. Addressing deficiencies of various substances improves overall resistance to disease.

The older person in the second example needs to improve circulation and, in part, to reverse processes which lead to deterioration. Plant extracts such as Ginkgo biloba improves efficiency and function of tissues subject to sub-optimal circulation. Niacin increases blood flow via dilation of blood vessels and may restore cholesterol to a more optimal state. Turmeric (Curcuma longa) reduces the tendency to build-up of blockages within the walls of arteries, and helps prevent deterioration of tissues. Various substances help prevent tissue deterioration and foster repair. Optimal repair of nerve tissue needs an abundance of the components found in such tissue cofactors which make them work. Lecithin contains materials needed for cell wall repair, and chemicals needed for communication between nerve cells. Vitamin B12, alpha-lipoic acid, and thiamin are co-factors that help maintain and repair nerve tissue. Various nutritional substances help to directly remove toxins, or fortify the detoxification organs of the body so they are more effective in achieving their intended purpose. Adequate detoxification is necessary for normal function and repair. Vitamin C, garlic, and chlorella, are helpful. And many nutritional substances have multiple benefits.

Animal and plant substances may be used in various ways. For example, extracts from fetal (unborn young) sheep tissues, such as from the fetal auditory nerve, may be taken by injection to stimulate organization and regeneration of human tissues associated with hearing. Fetal tissue is programmed by nature to generate into fully functioning organ systems. After peak reproductive years, bodily tissues are programmed to disorganize and deteriorate to eventually make room for the next generations to come. The use of fetal tissue appears, in part, to counter this trend.

The most important aspect of nutritional care in regard to ear problems lies between the ears in taking care of the needs of the rest of the person who is attached to the ears.

5. Most of us would assume, once hair cells die, the condition is permanent with irreversible sensorineural hearing loss. Would you share with readers what you've discovered, and any implications it might hold for restoration of hearing in humans?

Matthew Kelley, PhD is a Senior Investigator and Section Chief in the Intramural Program at the National Institute for Deafness and other Communication Disorders at NIH. He received a Ph.D. from the University of Virginia and was a Research Fellow at the University of Washington. His laboratory examines the genetic pathways that regulate the formation of mechanosensory hair cells within the mammalian cochlea.

Our sense of hearing is dependent on mechanosensory hair cells, microscopic sensory transducers located within the cochlea, which are able to transform sounds waves into nervous impulses that are interpreted by our brains as sound. While hearing loss can occur through several different mechanisms, death of mechanosensory hair cells is the most common reason. Unlike skin or muscle cells that are replaced when they're lost, in mammals mechanosensory hair cells are only produced during embryonic development, so as hair cells are lost in adults, a progressive and permanent hearing deficit will occur. Because hair cells are not replaced, research in my laboratory is focused on identifying the genetic pathways that direct a cell to develop as a hair cell. Since this only happens during embryonic development, we use the developing mouse embryo as a model system. Figure 3-1 shows an image of hair cell stereociliary bundles in the cochlea of a normal mouse. Four rows of mechanosensory hair cells are present. Each hair cell has a stereociliary bundle. Note a bright white arch "⌒" (see arrows) on its surface.

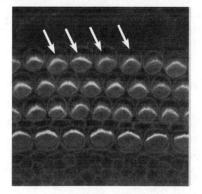

Figure 3-1: hair cell stereociliary bundles in the cochlea of a normal mouse

Recently, the work of several laboratories, including mine, have identified a particular gene that seems to play a crucial role in hair cell formation and may hold the key to inducing at least some hair cell restoration in the inner ear. Transcription factors are a kind of protein that act to turn on other genes. Therefore, these types of proteins are often able to direct significant changes in cells, like directing cells to become a particular type of cell. Several years ago, molecular genetic techniques were used to generate a family of mice in which the transcription factor, Atonal Homolog 1 (Atoh1 for short) was removed (Figure 3-2).

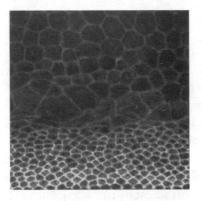

Figure 3-2: mouse cochlea where Atoh1 gene has been removed

An examination of the cochleas from these mice indicated that all of the hair cells were completely absent. However, perhaps a more exciting result was obtained several years later when cells within the inner ear that normally would not express Atoh1 were forced to express Atoh1 using molecular genetic techniques. Surprisingly, expression of Atoh1 appeared to make these cells develop as hair cells. In these experiments, hair cells formed in regions of the inner ear where hair cells normally would not be present and so it was unlikely that these cells would actually help to restore hearing, but more recent experiments have either forced expression of Atoh1 using a form of gene therapy or used pharmacological treatments to block a pathway that apparently actively prevents Atoh1 expression in the ears of adult animals that were recently deafened. While not every animal in these experiments experienced a recovery, some of them did, suggesting the modulation of this transcription factor may lead to the formation of new hair cells.

Similarly, in a scientific paper published in 2007, researchers at Kansas State University demonstrated a recovery of chemically induced balance disorders in guinea pigs in which Atoh1 was expressed in the inner ear using gene therapy. Our sense of balance is also controlled in our inner ear and depends on the presence of functional hair cells. An examination of the ears from these animals indicated that some new hair cells had been generated as a result of the Atoh1 gene therapy. Together, these findings provide strong evidence that Atoh1 is a crucial gene for the formation of hair cells and that using gene therapy to force expression of Atoh1 or eliminating a natural inhibitor of Atoh1 can lead to some new hair cells and some recovery of function in adult animals. However, there are a number of hurdles that must be cleared before we will be ready to try to treat human deafness or even balance disorders with Atoh1. First and foremost, recovery of function was not observed in every animal in any of these experiments, and in many cases the recovery that was observed was modest. Still, the discovery of Atoh1 as a factor that can make cells become hair cells and the demonstration that it can be used to produce some functional recovery in the inner ear is very exciting and suggests that researchers are on the right track to identify the genetic pathways that will lead to hair cell regeneration.

6. In light of current research, what advice can you offer the concerned consumers about recreational noise?

Brian Fligor, PhD is an audiologist and Director of Diagnostic Audiology at Boston Children's Hospital, and is on faculty at Harvard Medical School in the department of Otology and Laryngology. His work on recreational noise-induced hearing loss, particularly from headphones, has received considerable media attention and helped shape recommendations set by the European Union's 2008 report on hearing loss risk and prevention from personal music players. He is author of the chapter "Recreational Noise" in The Consumer Handbook on Hearing Loss and Noise (in Chasin, ed, Auricle Ink Publishers, 2010).

We live in a noisy world! This may sound contrite, but the reality is that the world today is more heavily populated, and more densely populated than at any previous point in human history. This high population density coupled with all the technology that makes developed nations engines of economic prosperity has had a casualty: natural quiet. According to , acoustic ecologist and Emmy Award-winning sound recording engineer, time-intervals that are free of human-made noise for 15-minutes or more (that is, "natural quiet") no longer exist east of the Mississippi river. In 1984, Mr. Hempton documented 21 places in Washington state that met this stringent definition of "natural quiet." In 2007, only three of these places still had natural quiet for 15 minutes or longer.

As such, noise is ubiquitous in our lives. Mainly, noise sources that affect us all are transportation noise: car, train, and air travel. The World Health Organization has defined appropriate quiet as being under 55 dB (A-weighted) during night and 65 dBA during the day (reflecting the need for noise levels to be low enough for sleep during the night and low enough during the day for communication). In Europe, 40 percent of the population are exposed to continuous noise in excess of the night-time recommendation, and 20 percent are exposed to continuous noise in excess of the daytime recommendation. In New York City, sound levels in Time Square and Union Square do not drop below 70 dBA at any time; often, the cacophony is continuous at levels over 80 dBA due to heavy traffic. On the New York City subway, the average levels are 86 dBA (and levels range between 84-112 dBA). One study indicated that a small but substantial percent of NYC subway users will lose a little hearing as a result of a lifetime of riding the subway.

Given the intrusion of noise made by others, many of us choose to take control of our own "soundscape." We do this in the form of listening to music on car stereos or (more commonly since the invention of MP3 players) on portable digital music players, like the iPod. The ability to escape the uncontrollable sounds of the city, avoiding (i.e., acoustically covering up) car alarms, subway noise, car horns, and being asked for money or directions is a reason sociologists have called the iPod the "urban Sherpa." Consequently, there is good evidence that people are listening to headphones louder and longer than at any previous time. While the majority of people do use their headphones safely, a substantial minority are at risk for noise-induced hearing loss. Such hearing loss develops insidiously; no measurable hearing loss occurs until at least five years of loud and protracted music listening, even in the most tender-eared listeners. Many people won't experience noise-induced hearing loss until 15-20 years of exposures, simply because their genetics give them "tougher ears" than average. This variability in susceptibility to noise-induced hearing loss has long been known, and creates a real challenge to hearing healthcare professionals in sending a unified message of "how loud and how long is too loud for too long?" The problem is, this cut-off for safe versus unsafe listening actually varies from one person to the next. In an effort to offer at least a general guideline that is perhaps slightly over-protective, but relatively permissive nonetheless, some hearing health researchers have offered the "80-for-90" rule: it's okay to listen to an iPod (using the headphones that come with the device) at 80 percent of the maximum volume (i.e., 100 percent is "all the way up" on the volume dial) for 90-minutes per day or less (7 days per week) without increasing the risk for noise-induced hearing loss. This "80-for-90" was based on output levels from a large sample of headphones (not just iPods, but certainly included this most popular brand) and comparing this to various standards known for predicting different degrees of noise-induced hearing loss.

But headphones aren't the only culprit contributing to risk for noise-induced hearing loss. Without question, the number one cause of recreational noise-induced hearing loss is firearms exposure. Gun ownership is a right held sacred by a huge population in the United States, and by far, the vast majority of gun owners are responsible about safely storing and using their weapons. However, "safety" does not always extend to "hearing safety" in gun owners. A survey of over 36,000 children and adults aged 11-45 years asked questions about sound exposures, and included the question, "Have you fired a gun in the past year?" Forty to forty-five percent of men and boys said that they had, while 19-32 percent of women and girls said that they had fired a gun in the past year. A 2002 study of hearing protection use among hunters in Michigan reported that while half of them had learned about use of hearing protection (e.g., earplugs) in their firearms safety courses, only 12 percent used earplugs while hunting. This is consequential, because gunshots are the loudest sound most people ever hear: from small pistols to high caliber rifles and large bore shotguns, peak sound levels range from 140-174 dB. The previous issue of "how loud and how long" dictating risk for hearing loss with, for instance, music listening, is out the window with sounds this loud. Immediate permanent hearing loss occurs, no matter how short the exposure, when the ear receives 140 dB peak sound level. In highly susceptible individuals, this critical level for immediate damage might be as low as 132 dB. Thus, no gunshot is safe if taken without some form of hearing protection.

Other sources of recreational noise sufficient to put one's hearing at risk include woodworking (tools emit 60-111 dBA, with most tools above 80 dBA), attending NASCAR and other motorized sports (levels are 101-106 dBA), attending music concerts (average levels are 104 dBA), attending dance clubs (104-112 dBA), and even some noisy children's toys (peak levels for some toys exceed 120-138 dBA when held at the ear, which some children do).

The number one thing a person can do to limit noise-induced hearing loss risk is to respect your hearing: use earplugs when you have to shout over the noise to be heard; if you can't use earplugs, walk away from the loud sound; give yourself quiet breaks if your ears sound muffled or you have ringing after a loud exposure. These actions translate into healthier behaviors for people who look to you for advice and guidance—your children. They imitate our behaviors, whether it's how we eat, how we exercise, or how we respect our ears (or don't). Hearing is a gift to be enjoyed for as long as possible.

7. From your research, what have you discovered about the process of listening?

Richard D. Halley, PhD is Emeritus Professor of Communication at Weber State University, Ogden, Utah, and considered an expert on the topic of listening. He has been a longtime board member of the International Listening Association, serving as its president, and has written many papers and a few books on the subject matter. Among newsworthy attention directed to Dr. Haley's work, he has been a repeated guest on ABC's "20/20."

The most obvious connection between hearing and listening is that if one does not hear the sounds, we cannot expect that person to interpret the meaning of the sounds with any accuracy. One of the things we know about listening is that people tend to hear what they want to hear (or more accurately what they expect to hear). Each individual literally creates in their mind a fairly accurate mathematical model of what they expect a message to be like. This capacity makes it possible for listeners to predict something about what a person is likely to say.

The advantage is that often when we're listening and we don't hear a small part of a sentence, we can guess rather accurately at what the rest of the sentence is. However, if you lose some hearing, you still have the mathematical models in your head and the predictions for what comes next in a message remain pretty strong. Yet, if you're not hearing accurately or are missing some of the sounds (some of the words even), your capacity to accurately predict is greatly reduced. If we hear accurately one word or phrase, we can do a reasonable job of predicting what the next word or phrase might be within some learned probability. At least we can narrow it down to just a few options. However, if we do not hear that word or phrase accurately, then we will make our prediction based on that inaccurate information and have a strong tendency to guess the next word or phrase inaccurately. And as we continue to listen, the problem gets compounded.

If you have a hearing loss, you must learn to be conscious of the effects it has on your ability to predict. If you're careful, prediction can help you understand because your brain often knows how to fill in some of the missing parts. But if you assume your processes of assigning meaning are still as accurate as they were before your hearing loss, and you interpret messages based on what was misheard (as certainly you will), the number of interpretation errors you make will increase dramatically.

One of the things we know is that men and women process information differently. Thus, it's important that we not talk as though all of our advice will work exactly the same for both sexes. One of the major differences is that, in general, most men are better than most women at staying focused on one speaker and ignoring others in the environment. This has the advantage that many men may be able to work in situations that are noisier than many women can tolerate. It has the significant disadvantage that men often don't hear someone call to them when they're concentrating on a message such as a television program, or more specifically, like Monday night football! This is true for men with good hearing. If you're hard of hearing, listening becomes that much more difficult. You might not hear a major portion of a message because you didn't switch to the new sound stream quickly enough and thus interpretations of the meaning of the message can be very inaccurate.

For example, let's suppose a wife says to her husband while he's watching a football game on television, "Honey, will you set the table? Dinner will be ready in 15 minutes." If the husband doesn't make the focus and listening switch until the word "table," all he'll likely process is something about "dinner" and "15 minutes." so he's very likely to continue watching the football game. Later there will be an interchange about "Why isn't the table set?" and the husband will be certain that he was not asked to set the table. If the husband had the most common type of hearing loss (for high frequency sounds), this message would be even more difficult regardless of the point at which the switch to the wife's message was made. It should be noted that many times a husband in this situation, with hearing loss and environmental noise that cancels out the message, might miss the entire communication altogether. Should this happen, he'll be mystified about even having been spoken to about dinner! Thus, accurate interpretation of the meaning is quite difficult.

On the other hand, women far more often than men tend to check their environment for other important messages. The advantage is that women can often work on one task and be able to check another task often enough that they can also complete the second task. For example, many women can fix dinner or work on some other task while staying aware of a small child without putting the youngster at risk. Their multi-focus ability exceeds that of men. The disadvantage is that when women listen to a message that requires a great deal of concentration (perhaps because the material is new or difficult), they will still check their environment for other mes-sages and may miss critical parts of that difficult message, and thus become confused or misunderstand the message. As hearing deteriorates, more parts of the "switched to message" are missed, and thus interpretation of the messages meaning is negatively affected.

So, listening requires focus despite your gender, and whether you have good hearing or not. Hearing loss merely makes the listening process more challenging.

8. In what ways do you believe baby boomers might impact hearing healthcare?

Nancy Kent has over 20 years' experience in marketing strategy, and is President of Mindshare Creative, a full-service marketing communications firm based in Southern California. Previously Ms. Kent was President of Primelife, a marketing agency that specialized in creating uniquely effective marketing programs for companies with products or services targeting consumers age 40 and older.

As they have influenced almost every aspect of society throughout their lives, the boomers will significantly impact hearing healthcare as they age. As the data reveals, there are more than 30 million people today with hearing loss. That number is expected to significantly grow as the boomers continue to age. Today, baby boomers are already impacting hearing healthcare as patients and caregivers. As more boomers begin to experience age-related hearing loss, they'll seek products or services that enable them to live youthful, active and social lives. Also, a significant number of boomers are part of the "Sandwich Generation"—a caregiver responsible for both aging parents and children. As the caregiver they're either the decision-maker or an influencer when it comes to their parent's hearing healthcare decisions.

To better understand what the boomers will be like as they age, we need to take a look back to the events that occurred while they were growing up, during their formative young adult years. The first of the boomers came of age in 1963, during a very turbulent time in our country. They experienced Vietnam and the Kennedy and King assassinations. They also grew up in an age of economic prosperity. The late boomers' formative years were highlighted by the end of the Vietnam conflict, Watergate, the Arab Oil Embargo and a faltering economy.

The events of the boomer's formative years created two attitudes that are important to hearing health professions. First, both segments of the baby boom generation are self-focused and are committed to maintaining their youth. We can expect this focus to become even stronger as boomers continue to age. Unfortunately, there are some significant indications that because of their high stress lifestyle, the boomers are not aging as well as they would like. In the federally funded Health and Retirement Study, boomers were much less likely than previous generations to describe their health as "excellent" or "very good." And, when it comes to hearing health, the years of enjoying rock and roll music are taking their toll. The 2006 Foundation and Clarity Study found 53 percent of baby boomers are already reporting at least "mild" hearing loss.

Second, both segments have a "debt imprint," which they will keep for life. For the Early boomers, the economy's strength manifested an optimistic attitude. They've saved little for retirement and are comfortable using credit to fund the lifestyle they desire. The Late boomers saw the S&P lose 30 percent of its value during their formative years. Debt became a way of life. And unlike the older boomers, the younger boomer's dependence on credit wasn't because they believed that times would always be good, but because they just assumed they could always get additional credit. For both segments of the baby boomers, paying with credit will always be their preference. Even today, healthcare professionals are adding payment plans when buying hearing aid to meet the expectations and desires of boomers.

Because of their self-focus, boomers will begin eliminating the social stigma that surrounds hearing aids. They have always considered themselves "hip" and will not let aging change that self-perception. Boomers will be unwilling to minimize their activities to accommodate their hearing loss, so a larger percentage of the group will readily accept hearing aid technology. In fact, the Foundation and Clarity 2006 Hearing Loss Study found that "Boomers, generally speaking, are willing to admit to having a hearing loss." As a significant portion of baby boomers become hearing aid wearers, the majority will rule and the stigma will begin to be minimized.

Throughout their lives baby boomers have enjoyed being the focus of marketers and businesses. As they begin to enter into retirement, they'll begin redefining aging. Hearing healthcare providers who choose to actively target boomers and effectively communicate with them will realize the potential that this large population segment represents. And we may see the primary barriers to purchasing hearing aids change as aging—and hearing technology—become hip and trendy.

9. Most people have heard of the condition known as Ménière's disease, but few, including those suffering from it, have a good understanding of the problem. Can you help clarify this disorder, and how it might differ from the similar condition of labyrinthitis?

Dennis Poe, MD, PhD is an otolaryngologist specializing in neurotologic surgery at the Massachusetts Eye and Ear, Boston, and is Editor of, and Contributor to *The Consumer Handbook on Dizziness and Vertigo* (Auricle Ink Publishers, 2005). Dr. Poe is a Past-Board member of the Prosper Ménière's Society and considered a foremost expert on Ménière's Disease.

Dizziness and balance disorders are very common and rank among the most frequent problems seen on a daily basis by health care providers of all types. The most common causes of sudden vertigo or imbalance are Vestibular Neuritis, an inflammation or irritation of the balance nerve, labyrinthitis, inflammation or irritation of the inner ear, Migraines, causing reduced blood flow to the balance centers in the brain, and Ménière's disease, a disruption of the inner ear due to fluid swelling. Labyrinthitis and Ménière's disease may be associated with varying degrees of hearing loss.

Medical professionals define vertigo as any hallucination of movement when in fact no real movement has occurred. The most common form of this is the spinning sensation that results after rapidly rotating oneself and stopping quickly. If vertigo is severe enough, it can cause secondary symptoms of nausea, vomiting, and cold sweats. It's estimated that about one third of the population will experience a significant bout of sudden vertigo during their lifetime, and the vast majority of these are due to vestibular neuritis or labyrinthitis. Still, Ménière's is common enough to affect as many as one out of 50 individuals.

Vestibular neuritis is presumably caused by viral inflammation of the vestibular (balance) nerve that brings inner ear information to the brain and results in vertigo and balance disturbances without hearing loss. More severe cases may also damage hearing or the cochlear nerve. Viral inflammation of the inner ear itself is called labyrinthitis and usually causes both vertigo and hearing loss. Severe cases of neuritis or labyrinthitis can cause sudden unexpected vertiginous attacks with a complete loss of balance that is made worse by any head movements or by watching anything move.

These symptoms can often last for hours causing nausea, vomiting, sometimes diarrhea, all of which can be a profoundly frightening experience. The episodes are usually quite harmless and completely resolve on their own in a few days without any treatment. Like many viral illnesses, it normally will not recur. More severe forms may cause a few after shock spells of lesser magnitude within a few days of the original attack. Once the acute vertigo attacks have subsided, there's a period of dysequilibrium—a sensation that the balance is off, and may last for hours, days, or many weeks, depending on the severity of the attacks. Treatment is usually limited to symptom relief with medications to quiet the balance system. A regular exercise program is recommended to speed up the recovery process after the balance injury by stimulating the natural process of *vestibular compensation*.

Even if some degree of permanent injury were to have occurred, the brain can use information from the injured balance organ or nerve and combine it with information from the normal side. The new balance signals are integrated with the vision and senses of position and feeling in the limbs to recreate an effective balance system. Exercising speeds up this compensation process.

Ménière's disease is believed to be the long-term result of an injury to the labyrinth, such as severe labyrinthitis that has failed to heal properly and has gone on to become a recurring cause of vertigo attacks and hearing injury. Symptoms of Ménière's Disease include recurring vertigo attacks, fluctuating hearing loss, abnormal noises in the ear (tinnitus), and pressure or fullness in the ear. This can be caused by a condition known as endolymphatic hydrops (swelling of the endolymph). This is the fluid that fills the innermost compartment of the inner ear. The excessive pressure is believed to result from a breakdown in the pressure-regulating mechanisms and can be simplistically likened to water on the knee years after an injury. When the inner ear fluids swell, it causes some strain that initially may be mistaken for pressure in the middle ear, as might be experienced with infections, or airplane travel. If the swelling continues, hearing loss, especially in the lower frequencies, may fluctuate and be associated with tinnitus, the warning noises the ear creates when injured.

Ultimately, unprovoked episodes of spinning vertigo can develop, sometimes even waking someone from sleep with a violent sense of rotation, nausea, and vomiting. The attack can last for minutes or hours and usually subsides, leaving the person exhausted and very unstable with significant dysequilibrium for many more hours, days, or even weeks, going through the same vestibular compensation recovery as occurs after a labyrinthitis spell.

Ménière's is much more disabling because these spells recur unexpectedly and with variable frequency, creating a tremendous loss of confidence in oneself. If the vertigo attacks occur frequently enough, there may be insufficient time between spells for vestibular compensation to occur and the person will experience chronic dysequilibrium with intermittent vertigo attacks, never having a chance to fully recover. Healthcare professionals and patients have difficulty sorting out the difference between spontaneous vertigo attacks, and the head movement or position-induced vertigo and dysequilibrium during the compensation phase.

In its early stages, Ménière's disease can be exceedingly difficult to diagnose but early recognition and treatment may be useful in arresting the progression of the disease from its natural course of hearing and balance degeneration. Each time a hydrops (accumulation of fluid) episode occurs, it does a small amount of cumulative permanent damage to the inner ear.

Treatment for Ménière's disease is directed toward controlling the endolymphatic fluid swelling since in 90 percent of patients no active cause will be identified. The body uses sodium as its principal regulator of fluid balance, so a strict 2000-milligram daily sodium-restricted diet is recommended. A sodium guidebook is recommended to learn about packaging labels and natural sodium content in foods. Simply removing the saltshaker from the table is inadequate to treat this disorder and strict regular adherence to a 2000 mg diet is strongly recommended while symptoms are active. Most people who do adhere to their diet notice a substantial difference when they eat out and cannot control their sodium intake, experiencing more symptoms within one or two days afterwards.

The second most important factor in controlling Ménière's is controlling stress. The hormonal release associated with stress has a profound effect on aggravating Ménière's disease, although, the mechanism for this is poorly understood. It's quite obvious that an increase in spells occurs during times of crises, injury, or illness. Gaining emotional control over Ménière's disease is a critical issue in preventing oneself from falling into the trap of becoming a victim to the condition. Victims live in the constant fear that an attack may occur, and the very stress of this fear actually creates more attacks. Many people who understand this situation find that they can exert their will over spells, and sometimes avert them. Caffeine, nicotine, and other powerful stimulants have also been known to aggravate Ménière's. Decaffeinated beverages and cessation of smoking are always recommended.

Physicians will often add a diuretic (water pill) to the treatment regimen to reduce the inner ear fluid pressure. Diuretics are often used for several months, and discontinued if the condition can be controlled by diet alone. If the spells cannot be adequately managed, then vestibular suppressants are often prescribed. These medications are all central nervous system depressants in nature, trying to slow down the abnormal impulses within the balance system, or anti-nausea medications that also help stabilize balance. Such medications are for symptom assistance only and do not prevent vertigo attacks. They may be used on a daily, even round-the-clock basis for short periods of time.

Medical treatment for Ménière's is generally successful in controlling the attacks, limiting them to one or two significant attacks per year, and most people don't require surgery. About 20 percent of Ménière's patients ultimately fail medical treatment and desire surgical intervention to stop the vertiginous attacks. Most of the procedures are designed to deaden the affected balance nerve so that the abnormal imbalance signals no longer reach the brain, and the vertigo attacks cease. Newer less invasive treatments are being developed but remain investigational. When there are no further disturbances in the balance system, vestibular compensation can occur as the opposite inner ear adjusts to the new balance arrangement.

10. Cochlear implants have been around now for a number of years. As an expert on this, can you tell us what a cochlear implant is, who is a candidate and the latest achievements in this area?

William Luxford, MD is a physician at the House Ear Clinic in Los Angeles, and Clinical Associate Professor of Otolaryngology at the University of Southern California School of Medicine. He has been performing implant surgeries for years and is extensively published in this area.

In general, cochlear implant candidates have a bilateral severe-profound sensorineural hearing loss, receive little or no benefit from conventional hearing aids, are in good physical and mental health, and have the motivation and patience to complete a rehabilitation program. A cochlear implant is an electronic prosthetic device that is surgically placed in the inner ear, under the skin behind the ear to provide sound perception to selected severe-to-profound hearing-impaired individuals (Figure 3-3).

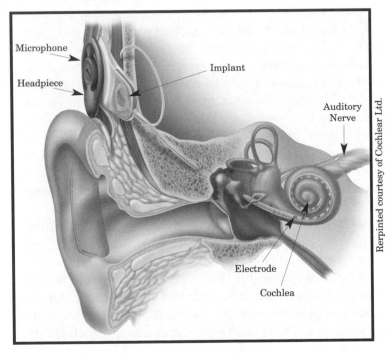

Figure 3-3: illustration of a cochlear implant

In addition to the internal component of the system, the cochlear implant has external parts that are worn outside the ear, including the microphone, speech processor, headpiece antenna and cable. A cochlear implant is NOT a hearing aid. A hearing aid amplifies acoustic signals, thereby making sounds louder and clearer to the person with hearing loss. Hearing aid-amplified acoustic signals are delivered to the ear and converted into electrical impulses by hair cells of the inner ear in exactly the same manner as sounds that are transmitted to the normal hearing ear.

A cochlear implant, on the other hand, converts acoustic sound vibrations into electrical signals, which are then coded and patterned in a manner designed to enhance speech perception. Through an externally worn antenna and internally implanted receiver, these coded electrical signals are then transmitted to an electrode in the inner ear which directly stimulates the auditory nerve fibers, thus bypassing the damaged hair cells of the cochlea. The electrical impulses are delivered to the brain where they are interpreted as meaningful sounds.

Potential candidates for cochlear implants include both children and adults with a wide age range. For the most part, children are at least 12-months old, while there are many people in their 80s who are successful users. Candidates undergo a very thorough evaluation, including medical, audiological and radiological assessment. The medical evaluation includes a complete history and physical examination to detect problems that might interfere with the patient's ability to complete either the surgical or rehabilitative measures of implantation. In adults, the cause of deafness would not seem as important as its onset. Adults who become deaf later in life, and who have fully developed speech and language before losing their hearing, are able to make better use of the implant than those who are born deaf or lose their hearing very early in life. On the other hand, the prelingually deafened child, if implanted early in life, can receive a great deal of benefit from a cochlear implant.

Counseling is important so that the patient and the family will have realistic expectations regarding benefits and limitations. Support from family and friends is essential in the rehabilitative process. The definition of success is different from person to person, and family to family. Memory of sound appears to be one of the most important factors for success in adults. Early implantation, and placement in an educational program that emphasizes development of auditory skills appear to be important factors for success in children.

Initially, only those patients who were stone deaf in both ears were considered implant candidates. With significant improvements in implant technology and signal processing, the benefits gained by implanted patients, both children and adults, have markedly improved. These improvements have led to a broadening of the criteria for implant patients. Selected patients with severe hearing loss receiving some benefit from appropriately fitted hearing aids are now considered possible implant candidates. Hearing aid technology has also improved. Most likely, patients with mild and moderate hearing loss will be candidates for hearing aids. Patients with severe loss will be candidates for either a hearing aid or cochlear implant, depending upon how well they function with the appropriate device. Patients with profound hearing loss will probably receive the best benefit through the use of a cochlear implant.

CHAPTER FOUR

Hearing Aids Can Transform Your Life

Sergei Kochkin, PhD

Dr. Kochkin is past Executive Director of the Better Hearing Institute (Washington, DC). He has 25 years of corporate experience as a market researcher and industrial psychologist. He has published close to 100 papers on the hearing loss population and the hearing aid market and conducted extensive customer satisfaction research on more than 35,000 hearing aid owners. He holds a doctorate in psychology, a MBA in marketing, a Master's of Science in counseling and guidance, and a BA in physical anthropology and archaeology. Dr. Kochkin also maintains an interest in ancient cultures, comparative religion, meditation, and golf.

People purchase their first hearing aids usually because they've recognized that their hearing has worsened. In other words, some critical incident in their life has caused them to realize that their hearing loss was negatively impacting their life or the life of a loved one. Some finally realized that they were missing the finer aspects of life such as music, the softly voiced communication from their grandchildren, or the ability to comprehend what was going on at social gatherings or at the theater. They often found themselves being left behind socially, and becoming more and more isolated from shared experiences. On the job, some experienced underperformance and being passed over for promotions and salary increases. Baby boomers on the dating scene in their 1950s have found themselves challenged in meaningful conversation, underpinning many relationship failures.

Furthermore, some caregivers endanger their grandchildren because denial of hearing loss puts them at risk. Untreated hearing loss can be life threatening when you consider that some sounds in life warn us of danger, such as smoke and carbon monoxide detectors, car horns, sirens and even the sound of the garbage disposer. I'm aware of a woman with hearing aids who got them only after she damaged her hand pushing garbage into the garbage disposal not knowing it was running. A second reason people try hearing aids is that they feel pressure from family members negatively impacted by the individual's hearing loss. Family members find it exhausting to be the ears for their loved one in denial, and finally after long years of frustration and countless arguments, the individual visits a hearing health professional.[1-5]

As you know by now, hearing loss occurs gradually. By the time you recognize a need for hearing aids, whether because you have come to that realization on your own or others have pushed you to it, your quality of life may have unnecessarily deteriorated. Although the majority (60 percent) of people with hearing loss are below the age of 65 and 36 percent of all people with hearing loss are below the age of 55, the average first-time hearing aid wearer is close to 70 years of age.[1]

The vast majority of individuals have decided to wait to correct their faulty hearing with hearing aids. This comprises 75 percent of all people who admit to hearing loss and 60 percent of people with moderate-severe hearing loss (and only 9 percent of people with mild hearing loss). I suspect that while they may be aware their hearing has deteriorated, they delay hearing aid purchases with the excuses: "My hearing loss is not bad enough yet; I can get by without them; my hearing loss is mild." Yet half of these people report they've never had their hearing professionally tested, had their hearing last checked as a child or more than 10 years earlier.[2]

A large number of people wait 15 years or more from the point when they first recognize they have a hearing loss to when they purchase their first hearing aids. This is a tragedy because they might not be aware of the impact this delayed decision has had on their life and the lives of their family, friends and associates. Yet, when people finally realize the extent of their hearing loss and understand the impact that hearing loss has on their life, the average person acts rationally, correcting their hearing loss with hearing aids within 3 years (median average) of diagnosis.[1]

So for most people with hearing loss, it's an issue of awareness: understanding the extent of their hearing loss and comprehending the impact that hearing loss has on their quality of life. Let's now review the literature on the impact of hearing loss on quality of life.

Hearing Loss and Quality of Life

The literature presents a compelling story of the social, psychological, cognitive and health effects of hearing loss. Impaired hearing results in distorted or incomplete communication, leading to greater isolation and withdrawal and therefore reduced sensory input. In turn, the individual's life space and social life become restricted. One would logically think that a constricted life would negatively impact the psychosocial well-being of people with hearing loss.

Dr. Carmen presented a number of emotional issues in Chapter One surrounding hearing loss. Here's a quick review, with some additional ones. The literature associates hearing loss with embarrassment, fatigue, irritability, tension and stress, anger, avoidance of social activities, withdrawal from social situations, depression, negativism, danger to personal safety, rejection by others, reduced general health, loneliness, social isolation, less alertness to the environment, impaired memory, less adaptability to learning new tasks, paranoia, reduced coping skills, and reduced overall psychological health. For those who are still in the workforce, uncorrected hearing loss must have a negative impact on overall job effectiveness, promotion, and perhaps lifelong earning power. Few would disagree that uncorrected hearing loss per se is a serious issue.

Prior Experimental Evidence that Hearing Aids Improve Quality of Life

An effective human being is an effective communicator; critical to effective communication is optimized hearing. Modern hearing aids improve speech intelligibility and therefore communication. The benefits of hearing aids (audiologically defined as *improved speech intelligibility*) have been demonstrated in rigorous scientific research.[6] It would seem that if one could improve speech intelligibility by correcting for impaired hearing, one should observe improvements in the social, emotional, psychological, and physical functioning of the person with the hearing loss. To my knowledge, only a few studies to date have compared hearing aid owners to non-owners with known hearing loss. The majority of studies had small sample sizes and in general tended to confine themselves to U.S. male veterans. I want to first share these results with you before describing the exciting findings of a very large U.S. study I conducted in collaboration with the National Council on Aging in 1999 and a more recent study on the impact of hearing loss on household income and quality of life. Later on, I will prove there is a price for vanity!

Harless and McConnell[7] demonstrated that 68 hearing aid wearers had significantly higher self-concepts compared to a matched group of individuals who did not wear hearing aids. Dye and Peak[8] studied 58 male veterans pre- and post-hearing aid fitting and found significant improvement on memory tests. In the most rigorous controlled study to date, Mulrow, Aguilar and Endicott[9] studied 122 male veterans and 72 patients from primary care clinics. Half were randomly chosen and fitted with hearing aids, while the other half were not. After four months of comparing hearing aid wearers to the control group, the researchers found significant improvements with regard to emotional and social effects of hearing handicap, perceived communication difficulties, cognitive functioning, and depression.

In addition, the same researchers in a follow-up study[10] published in 1992 demonstrated that the quality of life changes were sustainable over at least a year. Bridges and Bentler[11] determined in a study of 251 subjects comprised of normal hearing elderly individuals with hearing aids and individuals with unaided hearing loss that hearing aid wearers had less depression and higher quality of life scores compared to their unaided counterparts.

Finally, in a pre-post study (that is, the person was studied before and after a hearing aid fitting) with 20 subjects, Crandall[12] demonstrated that after three months of hearing aid use, functional health status improved significantly for hearing aid wearers.

Research on the Positive Impact of Hearing Aids on Quality of Life

I would now like to share with you the results of the largest study in the world conducted on the impact of hearing aids on quality of life.[13-14] Reading this should persuade you that hearing aids successfully fit to your unique audiological needs have the potential to literally transform your life. Utilizing the famous National Family Opinion Panel (NFO) in 1997, I mailed a short screening survey to 80,000 panel members to find a representative sample of people with hearing loss in the United States. This short survey helped identify nearly 15,000 people with self-admitted hearing loss. The response rate to the screening survey was 65 percent. Since 1989, I've conducted research in this manner on more than 25,000 people with hearing loss and published these findings under the generic name "MarkeTrak." Working with the National Council on Aging, I drew a random sample of 3,000 individuals with hearing loss ages 50 and over from the MarkeTrak hearing loss panel. Equal samples of 1,500 hearing aid owners and non-owners were drawn from the panel.

What is unique about this study is that it studied people with hearing loss as well as their significant others (usually spouses).

Extensive questionnaires were sent to both the person with the hearing loss (300 questions) and the spouse or family member (150 questions). The comprehensive survey covered a myriad of topics: self and family assessment of hearing loss, psychological well-being, social impact of hearing loss, quality of relationships, life satisfaction, general health, self and family perceptions of benefit of hearing aids (wearers only), reasons for purchasing hearing aids (wearers only), reasons for not purchasing hearing aids (non-wearers only), and attitudes toward hearing health and hearing aids. In addition, the survey included a number of personality scales deemed relevant to this study.

After analyzing the returned surveys for usability and exclusions (such as for incompleteness of answers or respondents who failed to wear their hearing instruments), I reduced the final sample sizes to 2,069 for respondents with hearing loss, and to 1,710 for family members. Thus, this study involved nearly 4,000 people.

It was my goal to determine if hearing aids have an impact on hearing loss independent of the degree of hearing loss. In other words, do people with mild hearing loss derive as much benefit as individuals with more serious hearing loss? As part of the research design, in addition to quality of life items, I administered a paper and pencil assessment of hearing loss with the anticipation that the results of this assessment would control for hearing loss when comparing the quality of life of hearing aid wearers and non-wearers.

The key hearing assessment tool used was the *Five Minute Hearing Test* (FMHT) by the American Academy of Otolaryngology-Head and Neck Surgery (www.hearingcheck.org). This is a fifteen question test, measures self-perceived hearing difficulty in a number of listening situations (e.g., telephone, multiple talkers, television, noisy situations, reverberant rooms) as well as self-assessments of some signs of hearing loss (e.g., people mumble, inappropriate responses, strain to hear, avoid social situations). Previous research has significantly correlated the FMHT with objective audiological hearing loss measures.

Based on hearing difficulty scores, all subjects in this study were clustered into five groups of equal size (20 percent each—called quintiles). These ranged from quintile 1 (the 20 percent of respondents with the mildest hearing loss as measured by the FMHT) to quintile 5 (the 20 percent with the greatest hearing loss). The quintile system was utilized for all analysis as a means of controlling for differences in hearing loss between the hearing aid wearer and non-wearer samples. The use of these quintiles allowed us to achieve more valid comparisons between samples of hearing aid wearers and non-wearers.

If we had simply compared responses of all hearing aid wearers with those of all non-wearers, without regard to degree of hearing loss, the findings would have been misleading, and even erroneous. For example, it's widely known that incidence and degree of depression increase with severity of hearing loss. Thus, even if people with severe hearing loss experience reduced depression after getting hearing aids, they might still report more depression than non-wearers overall, because hearing aid wearers tend to have more severe hearing loss. However, when hearing aid wearers are matched with non-wearers in the same quintile (non-wearers having a fairly similar degree of hearing loss), the differences between them better reflect the potential impact of the hearing aids rather than the effect of their degree of hearing loss.

While we have no audiological basis for labeling hearing loss associated with each quintile group, we did find a meaningful correlation between self-perceived loss (e.g., mild to profound hearing loss) and the FMHT test. As we discuss the findings of this study with respect to the five hearing loss groups, it's appropriate to consider people in quintile hearing loss groups 1, 3, and 5 as having respectively a "mild," "moderate," and "severe /profound" hearing loss; group 2 is between mild and moderate hearing loss, while group 4 should be viewed as between moderate and severe hearing loss.

Research Findings

We will now systematically evaluate the impact that hearing aids have on quality of life by comparing the responses of hearing aid wearers and non-wearers while controlling for hearing loss. As you evaluate the impressive findings below, keep in mind the following:

- the devastating impact of hearing loss on quality of life is well-documented;
- quality of life is primarily impacted by the fact that uncorrected hearing loss results in reduced speech intelligibility;
- hearing aids, when fit correctly, improve speech intelligibility and therefore can restore your ability to function more effectively in life.

Hearing Less means Earning Less

In most respects the five hearing loss groups were well matched on key demographics: gender, marital status, employment status, and age. A striking trend was discovered when evaluating household income by level of hearing loss. Income significantly correlated to both hearing loss and hearing aid usage. We found a strong relationship between hearing loss and income: the greater the hearing loss, the greater the loss in income. More importantly, the use of hearing aids mitigated the impact of hearing loss on job performance as reflected in higher incomes for people who wore hearing aids on the job. Higher hearing disability levels probably impact communication, resulting in lower income and therefore less earning power. Finding a solution to their hearing loss is a problem exacerbated for people with hearing loss in the workforce because their lower earning power probably renders the respondents less able to afford a hearing aid to correct the hearing loss.

The trend correlating hearing loss with diminished income discovered in the NCOA study motivated me to investigate in more detail the impact of hearing loss on income in a large-scale study of nearly 40,000 households (published originally in 2007 and updated in 2010).[5] Before we continue with the groundbreaking NCOA study, it would be useful to review the results of this most recent study.

In November 2008, just prior to the publication of the third edition of this book, a short screening survey was mailed to 80,000 members of the National Family Opinion (NFO) panel. The NFO panel consists of households balanced to the latest U.S. census information with respect to market size, ages in a household, size of household, and income within each of the nine census regions, as well as by family versus non-family households. The screening phase identified close to 15,000 people with hearing loss as well as those who used hearing aids. Excluding children and people in the household who were not the head of household or spouse of the head of household, the following sample sizes were achieved for this study: <u>Aided</u>: 1,818 households where the head of household or spouse indicated that one or more had a hearing loss and that one or more wore a hearing instrument. <u>Unaided:</u> 3,232 households where neither the head of household nor spouse wore a hearing instrument but reported that one or more had a hearing loss. <u>Normal Hearing:</u> 34,351 households where the head or spouse did not report a hearing loss.

Because income was hypothesized to be related to degree of hearing loss based on the NCOA study, both aided and unaided subjects completed a battery of 28 questions related to the degree of their hearing loss. They were segmented into one of ten groups (called deciles) based on their responses to these questions, where a score of 1 means they had the mildest hearing loss (that is, they were in the lower 10 percent of people with hearing loss) and a 10 means they had the severest hearing loss (that is, they were in the top 10 percent of people with hearing loss). We have graphed the income differential (aided versus unaided) by degree of hearing loss (deciles) in Figure 4-1.

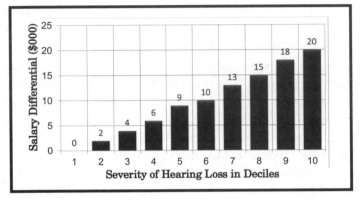

Figure 4-1: salary differential ($000) between aided and unaided) subjects by severity of hearing loss in deciles

The relationship we found is astounding and important information for all people with hearing loss. Regardless of whether hearing loss was mild, moderate or severe, we found a loss of income associated with hearing loss. Depending on degree of hearing loss, families are losing up to $31,000 per year in income depending on degree of hearing loss compared to normal hearing people. However, hearing aids mitigated the loss of income by about 90-100 percent for people with mild hearing loss, 77 percent for people with moderate hearing loss and 65 percent for people with severe hearing loss. Referring to Figure 4-1, the income gap between aided and unaided people grows dramatically from no difference in income at hearing loss decile 1 and $20,000 for people with severe hearing loss at decile 10. Taking into account the entire unaided hearing loss population, the estimated cost in lost earnings due to untreated hearing loss is $176 billion annually while the annual cost to society in terms of unrealized federal income taxes is $26 billion. Furthermore, people with hearing loss who used hearing aids on the job were 50 percent less likely to be unemployed.

Hearing is a critical sense for effective communication in the workforce. Most employment situations require verbal communication in order to effectively engage in commerce and deal with the public and fellow employees; appropriate hearing ability is also critical to assure safety on the job. Without aided hearing, as these data and the literature show, the person with hearing loss can be expected to suffer losses in compensation due to underemployment, may make mistakes on the job, may experience higher rates of unemployment, and in general may experience an overall reduction in quality of life (i.e., anxiety, depression, social isolation, social paranoia, medical health, emotional stability, cognitive functioning, etc.) which may negatively impact job performance.

Most hearing health professionals are aware of individuals who delayed hearing loss treatment well past their working lives due to fear of stigmatization on the job. This author is personally aware of a CEO who indicated that he had delayed treatment for his hearing loss due to vanity until a critical error caused him to lose a million dollar contract. We have also talked with individuals who suffered needlessly during their school years with "hidden" hearing loss. Unfortunately, untreated hearing loss is not actually hidden, since it results in underachievement for nearly all who delay treatment while they're in the prime of life. The tragedy is that untreated hearing loss impacts the individual and his or her family for the rest of his or her life in the form of lost wages, lost promotions, lost opportunities, and unrealized dreams, not to mention lower income in her or his retirement because of less discretionary income to save.

Now let's get back to the findings in other areas from the NCOA study.

Activity Level

We asked respondents to indicate the extent (times per month) to which they engaged in thirteen activities in a typical month. Six of the activities were solitary in nature while seven involved other people. Total solitary and social activity scores were calculated. Hearing aid wearers had the same level of solitary activity as non-wearers. However, hearing aid wearers were more likely to engage in activities involving other people. They had significantly higher participation in three to four of the seven activities measured. Four out of five quintile hearing aid wearer groups indicated they participated more in organized social activities while three out of five of the hearing loss groups reported they were more likely to attend senior centers if they were hearing aid wearers. The most serious hearing loss group (quintile 5) reported greater participation in four out of the seven activities if they were hearing aid wearers.

Interpersonal Relations

The survey, using a four-point scale for answers, asked 12 questions concerning the respondents' quality of interpersonal relationships with their family. Twelve questions concerned nega-tivity in the relationship (e.g., arguments, tension, criticism). As hearing loss worsened, interpersonal warmth in relationships significantly declined. Hearing aid wearers in quintiles 1-3 (mild to moderate) compared to their non-wearer counterparts had signifi-cantly greater interpersonal warmth in their relationships. Also, significant reductions in negativity in family relationships appeared to be associated with hearing aid usage in quintiles 1 and 2—the hearing loss groups with the mildest hearing disability.

Social Effects

Forty-seven items in the survey assessed the social impact of hearing loss and hearing aid usage. The majority of the items were scored on a five-point scale, taking the values "strongly agree" to "strongly disagree." We also assessed average monthly contact with family and friends by phone and in person.

As hearing loss increased, the fear of the stigma of hearing loss also increased. All five non-wearer groups reported they would feel embarrassed or self-conscious if they wore hearing aids, while all five wearer groups reported lower stigmatization with hearing aids. We're not concluding, of course, that usage of hearing aids would lead to reduced stigma; most likely, hearing aid wearers have resolved their concerns about the stigma associated with hearing aid usage, at least more so than their non-wearer counterparts.

As hearing loss increased, respondents were more likely to overcompensate for hearing loss by pretending that they heard what people said, by avoiding telling people to repeat themselves, by avoiding asking other people to help them with their hearing problem, by engaging in compensatory activities such as speechreading, or by defensively talking too much to cover up the fact that they couldn't hear well.

All five hearing aid wearer groups reported significantly lower overcompensation scores. The greater the hearing loss, the greater was the likelihood that respondents reported they were the target of discrimination. The greater the hearing loss, the greater was the likelihood that respondents with more serious hearing losses were accused of hearing only what they wanted to hear, found themselves the subject of conversation behind their backs, were told to "forget it" when they had not heard frustrated family members the first time, and so on. All hearing loss groups except quintile 1 (the mildest hearing loss) reported significant reductions in discriminatory behaviors, if they were hearing aid wearers.

We found a strong relationship between hearing loss and family member concerns of safety (e.g., cannot hear warning signs, missed instructions from doctor, made a serious mistake, is not safe to be alone) as well as significant differences between hearing aid wearers and non-wearers. Respondents also agreed that safety concerns increased as hearing loss increased.

The data, however, indicated that safety concerns were significantly higher among hearing aid wearers than non-wearers in quintiles 1-3. Perhaps the realization that mistakes were being made or that unaided hearing loss could result in possible injury motivated the current hearing aid owner to purchase hearing aids. This explanation is consistent with findings from previous MarkeTrak research, which indicated that the number one motivation to purchase hearing aids was "the realization that their hearing loss was getting worse."

A number of social effects correlated with hearing loss, but were not impacted by hearing aid usage. These were negative effects on the family (e.g., "I find it exhausting to cope with their needs"), family accommodations to the individual with hearing loss (e.g., "I have to use signs and gestures a lot of the time"), rejection of the person with hearing loss (e.g., "They tend to get left out of social activities because of their hearing loss"), and withdrawal (e.g., "They tend to withdraw from social activities where communication is difficult"). In addition, hearing aid usage was not associated with increased phone or in-person contact with family or friends.

The Emotional Effects

Eighty items in the survey dealt with the emotional aspects of hearing loss. All five hearing aid wearer groups scored significantly lower in their self-ratings of emotional instability. In agreement with their family members, they were less likely to be tense, insecure, unstable, nervous, discontented, or temperamental, and less likely to display negative emotions or traits. Four of the five hearing aid wearer groups reported significantly reduced tendencies to exhibit anger (e.g., "I sometimes get angry when I think about my hearing") and frustration (e.g., "I get discouraged because of my hearing loss"). In agreement, family members observed significantly less anger and frustration in all five hearing aid wearer groups.

The average reduction in depression associated with hearing aid usage across all five groups was 36 percent. All five hearing aid wearer groups reported significantly *lower* depressive symptoms (e.g., feeling tired, being insomniac, thinking of death) while four of the five hearing aid wearer groups (quintiles 1-4) reported a significantly lower incidence of depression within the last 12 months, compared to their non-wearer counterparts.

Hearing aid wearers in quintiles 2-4 reported significantly lower paranoid feelings (e.g., "I'm often blamed for things that are just not my fault"). Not surprisingly, in agreement with family members, all five non-wearer groups scored higher on denial when compared to hearing aid wearers (e.g., "I don't think my hearing loss is as bad as people have told me").

Family members and respondents indicated if the person with the hearing loss exhibited anxiety, showed tenseness, or worried for a continuous period of four weeks in the previous year. In addition, they indicated anxiety symptoms (e.g., being keyed up or on edge, heart pounding or racing, tiring easily, having trouble falling asleep). Three of the five non-wearer groups (1, 3, 5) exhibited higher anxiety symptoms. In addition, three of the five non-wearer groups (1, 2, 5) exhibited more social phobias than non-wearers of hearing aids. Clearly, the reduced phobia and anxiety associated with hearing aid usage are more pronounced in individuals with serious to profound hearing losses (quintile 5).

Factors *not* appreciably impacted by hearing aid usage in this study were sense of independence (e.g., burden on family, answering for the person with hearing loss) and overall satisfaction with life. Although not as conclusive as some of the previous factors, non-wearers reported that they were more self-critical (e.g., "I dwell on my mistakes more than I should") and had lower self-esteem (e.g., "All in all, I'm inclined to feel that I am a failure").

Personality Assessment

Seventy-nine items were devoted to miscellaneous personality scales in addition to the personality measures under emotional and social effects. All of the personality scales used in this study are published standardized scales. Family members indicated that the respondents' cognitive/mental state (e.g., they appear confused, disoriented, or unable to concentrate) was affected by degree of hearing loss, primarily if the hearing loss was "severe" to "profound" (groups 4 and 5) and the individual did not use hearing aids. In this study, impressive improvements in family perceptions of the persons' mental and intellectual state were observed if they wore hearing aids. Non-wearers were more likely to be viewed as being confused, disoriented, non-caring, arrogant or inattentive, and as virtually "living in a world of their own."

Previously we indicated that there were no significant differences in measures of withdrawal between aided and unaided subjects. This finding is contrary to the literature. However, family members did report that non-wearers in three of five groups (1, 4, 5) were more introverted as evidenced by greater likelihood of being private, passive, shy, quiet, easily embarrassed, etc. Moderate to severe hearing loss non-wearers (quintiles 3-5) scored higher on a personality variable called "external locus of control." This means they were more likely to believe that events external to them controlled their lives. In other words, they felt less in control of their own lives. On the other hand, hearing aid wearers felt they controlled more of their lives and were not as much victimized by fate.

Health Impact

The survey asked six generic questions on self-perceptions of health, prevalence of pain, and the extent to which the respondents believed that hearing loss impacted their general health. In addition, from a list of 28 health problems, respondents indicated whether they experienced that health problem and to what extent the problem interfered with their activities.

Overall assessment of health (including absence of pain) appeared to decline as a function of hearing loss with further deterioration of health associated with non-usage of hearing aids for the three most serious hearing loss groups (quintiles 3-5). Three of the five hearing aid wearer groups (quintiles 1, 3, 5) reported significantly better health compared to their non-wearer counterparts. The lowest self-rating of overall health was the non-wearer group in quintile 5 (profound hearing loss). Nonetheless, no consistent evidence associated hearing aid usage with reductions in arthritis, high blood pressure, heart problems, or other serious disease states.

Perceived Benefit of Hearing Aids

As a validation check on our comparisons of hearing aid wearers and non-wearers, both respondents and their family members rated changes they observed in 16 areas of their life that they believed were due to the respondents using hearing aids. Total findings are shown in Figure 4-2. In general, for nearly all quality of life areas assessed, the observed improvements positively related to degree of hearing loss. Family members in nearly every comparison observed greater improvements in the respondents than did hearing instrument wearers themselves.

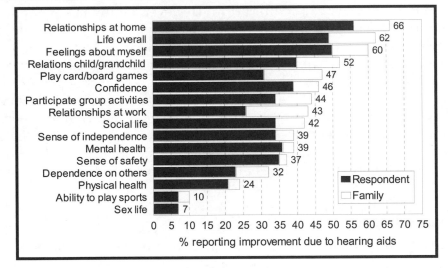

Figure 4-2: percent of hearing aid owners and their family members reporting improvement in their quality of life in 16 areas due to hearing aids

The top three areas of observed improvement for both respondents and family members were *relationships at home, feelings about self,* and *life overall.* The most impressive improvements were observed in quintile 5 (profound hearing loss) in that 11 of 16 lifestyle areas were rated as improved by at least 50 percent of the respondents or family members.

Hearing Handicap Reduction with Hearing Aids

By now you recognize that most people who have hearing loss experience problems associated with that hearing loss. If they did not experience problems in their quality of life then they would not need hearing aids or rehabilitative services. As a follow-up to the comprehensive NCOA study previously detailed we asked 1,871 hearing aid owners (with hearing aids 4 years old or less) to quantify the direct benefit they derived from their hearing aids.[15] Consumers were presented with ten listening situations and asked on a 0-100 percent scale to estimate the percent of their problem which was solved by use of hearing aids.

In Figure 4-3, the hearing handicap improvement is displayed in ten listening situations. Patients report a 70 percent improvement in quiet situations, and approximately a 60 percent improvement in small gatherings while on the phone and in a place of worship. Patients report about a 50 percent improvement in all other situations measured in this survey. In more detailed inquiry, nearly seven out of ten patients reported their ability to communicate effectively in most situations improved because of their use of hearing aids.

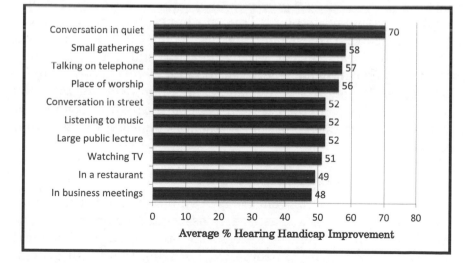

Figure 4-3: hearing handicap improvement (percent) for the U.S. population due to hearing aid usage in 10 listening situations (for hearing aids less than or equal to 4 years of age)

Slightly more than half of the patients reported hearing aids improved their relationships at home, their social life and their ability to participate in groups. Approximately four in ten reported improvements in: sense of safety, self-confidence, feelings about self, sense of independence and work relationships (for those working). Between a quarter and a third of respondents reported improvements in their sense of humor, mental and emotional health, romance, cognitive skills, and physical health. In assessing 14 quality of life areas, 75 percent of patients reported at least one area of their life had benefitted from hearing aid use. Additionally, eight out of ten were satisfied with the changes that had occurred in their lives due to hearing aids.

The results achieved by consumers of hearing aids will vary depending on the individual's degree of hearing loss, motivation, cognitive skills, use of assistive listening devices (such as wireless connection to your hearing aid), but most importantly based on the skill of the practitioner who fits the hearing aids. It's important to understand that you can ONLY achieve positive transformations in your life if you derive benefit from your hearing aids. Recent research has demonstrated that you are eight times more likely to get superb benefit from your hearing aids if the hearing health professional employs best practices then if they utilize a minimalist hearing aid fitting protocol.[15-16] Thus, it's imperative that you choose a hearing health professional with a good reputation and who employs best practices in fitting hearing aids. The potential consumer of hearing aids is advised to read *"Your Guide to Buying Hearing Aids"*[17] and to talk to friends and a family doctor to assure that you are referred to the best hearing healthcare professional. Dr. Sandlin's Chapter Eleven presents essential information on finding a practitioner.

Conclusions and Discussion

The impressive results from the NCOA, income studies and more recent studies on benefit, has clearly associated hearing aids with considerable improvements in the social, emotional, psychological, and physical well-being of people with hearing loss in all hearing loss categories from mild to severe. As such, these findings clearly provided strong evidence for the *value of hearing aids* in improving the quality of life in people with hearing loss. Specifically, hearing aid usage positively related to the following quality of life issues:

- greater earning power (especially the more severe hearing losses)
- improved interpersonal relationships (especially for mild-moderate losses) including greater intimacy and less negative dysfunctional communication
- reduction in discrimination toward the person with the hearing loss
- reduction in difficulty associated with communication (primarily severe to profound hearing losses)
- reduction in hearing loss compensation behaviors
- reduction in anger and frustration
- reduction in the incidence of depression and depressive symptoms
- enhanced emotional stability
- reduction in paranoid feelings
- reduced anxiety symptoms
- reduced social phobias (primarily severely impaired subjects)
- improved sense of control in your life
- reduced self-criticism
- improved cognitive functioning (primarily severe to profound hearing loss)
- improved health status and less incidence of pain
- enhanced group social activity

In the NCOA study, both respondents and their family members independently rated the extent to which they believed their life had specifically improved due to hearing aids. All hearing loss groups from mild to profound reported significant improvements in nearly every area measured:

- relationships at home and with family
- feelings about self
- life overall
- mental health
- social life
- emotional health
- physical health

A Call to Action

Dr. Firman of the National Council On Aging stated in his speech to the media in the summer of 1999, "This study debunks the myth that untreated hearing loss...is a harmless condition."[13]

In focus groups conducted with physicians, the prevalent view was that hearing loss is "only" a quality of life or benign issue. I would agree if one defined quality of life as "greater enjoyment of music." But the literature and this study clearly associated hearing loss with lessened physical, emotional, mental, and social well-being. Depression, anxiety, emotional instability, phobias, withdrawal, isolation, lessened health status, lower self-esteem, and so forth, are not "just quality of life issues." For some people, uncorrected hearing loss is a "life and death issue."

This study challenges every segment of society to comprehend the devastating impact of hearing loss on individuals and their families as well as the positive possibilities associated with hearing aid usage. We need to help physicians recognize hearing loss for the important health issue that it is. We need to help those with hearing loss currently in denial about their impairment to understand the impact their hearing has on their life as well as on their loved ones. We need to assure that society recognizes hearing aids not just as treatments for hearing loss, but also as potential contributors to the successful resolution of other medical, emotional, social and psychological conditions.

This study also demonstrates for the first time that individuals with even a mild hearing loss can experience dramatic improvements in their quality of life. This finding is significant because the challenge is to demonstrate to baby boomers (born 1946-1964) with emerging hearing losses that hearing aids offer something to them of such value that they do not need to wait until retirement to receive the benefits of enhanced hearing.

So if you're one of those people with a hearing loss who's sitting on the fence, consider all the benefits of hearing aids described in this book. Name another product that holds such great potential to positively change so many lives.

Editor's Note: The full research project this chapter is based on (including detailed references, charts and figures) is available at www.betterhearing.org under "Publications."[14]

References

1. Kochkin S. (2009). MarkeTrak VIII: 25 year trends in the hearing health market. *The Hearing Review,* Vol. 16 (11): 12-31.

2. Kochkin S. (2012). MarkeTrak VIII: The key influencing factors in hearing aid purchase intent. *Hearing Review.* 19 (3): 12-25.

3. Kochkin S. (2007). Is your child safe when grandpa can't hear? August, 2007: Retrieved from http://www.betterhearing.org/press/pdfs/naps_safety_publica ation.pdf.

4. Kochkin S. (2005). Hearing aids: an unexpected way to improve your sex life. Retrieved from http://deafness.about.com/od/hearing aids/a/bettersex.htm.

5. Kochkin S. (2010) The Efficacy of Hearing Aids in Achieving Compensation Equity in the Workplace, *The Hearing Journal,* 63 (10): 19-28.

6. Larson VD et al. (2000). Efficacy of three commonly used hearing aid circuits. *JAMA,* 284 (14):1806-1813.

7. Harless E & McConnell F. (1982). Effects of hearing aid use on self-concept in older persons. *Journal of Speech and Hearing Disorders,* 47: 305-309.

8. Dye C & Peak M. (1983). Influence on amplification on the psychological functioning of older adults with neurosensory hearing loss. *Journal of the Academy of Rehabilitation Audiology,* 16: 210-220.

9. Mulrow C, Aguilar C, Endicott J, et al. (1990).Quality of life changes and hearing impairment. *Annals of Internal Medicine,* 113 (3):188-194.

10. Mulrow C, Tuley M & Aguilar C. (1992). Sustained benefits of hearing aids. *Journal of Speech and Hearing Research,* 35: 1402-1405.

11. Bridges J & Bentler R. (1998). Relating hearing aid use to well-being among older adults. *The Hearing Journal,* 51 (7): 39-44.

12. Crandell C. (1998). Hearing aids: their effects on functional health status. *The Hearing Journal,* 51 (2): 2-6.

13. Firman J. (May 26, 1999). Speech to the media. Based on National Council on the Aging (NCOA). The impact of untreated hearing loss in older Americans. Conducted by the Seniors Research Group. Supported through a grant from the Hearing Industries Association. Preliminary report, December 28, 1998. Actual press release retrieved from http://www.ncoa.org.

14. Kochkin S and Rogin C. (2000). Quantifying the obvious: the impact of hearing aids on quality of life. *The Hearing Review,* 7 (1): 8-34.

15. Kochkin S. (2011). MarkeTrak VIII: Patients report improved quality of life with hearing aid usage, *Hearing Journal*, 64 (6): 25-32.

16. Kochkin S, Beck DL, Christensen, LA, et al. (2010). MarkeTrak VIII: The impact of the hearing healthcare professional on hearing aid user success, *The Hearing Review*, 17 (4): 12-34.

17. Kochkin, S. (2010). <u>Your Guide to Buying Hearing Aids</u>. Better Hearing Institute, Washington, D.C. See www.betterhearing.org under hearing loss treatment/hearing aids.

CHAPTER FIVE
Hearing Aid Technology and Rehabilitation

Robert W. Sweetow, PhD

Dr. Sweetow is a Professor of Otolaryngology in the Department of Otolaryngology at the University of California, San Francisco. He was the Director of Audiology at the UCSF Medical Center from 1991-2010. He received his PhD from Northwestern University in 1977, holds a Master of Arts degree from the University of Southern California, and a Bachelor of Science degree from the University of Iowa. Dr. Sweetow has lectured worldwide and has authored nearly 30 textbook chapters and over 120 scientific articles on counseling, tinnitus, aural rehabilitation and amplification for the hearing impaired. He is the co-developer of an interactive training program called Listening and Communication Enhancement (LACE) designed for home use.

Technological advances in hearing aids are progressing at an amazing pace. Similar to computers, the technology that was available as little as five years ago has now been replaced by more sophisticated hardware and software. Even so, many of the myths and misconceptions that were present five years ago regarding hearing aids still remain. The objective of this chapter is to prepare you with accurate up-to-date information to help in your decision to upgrade or try new hearing aids. Keeping up to date is very important, and sometimes difficult to do because technology is changing so rapidly. But in today's world, consumers need to be educated so that they can work together with their professional to make the best decisions possible. This chapter addresses questions you may ask yourself before and even during your test drive of hearing aids.

"Am I a candidate for hearing aids?"

Forty years ago, many hearing healthcare professionals believed that only people with hearing loss due to outer or middle ear problems (conductive hearing loss) could be helped by hearing aids. Patients were often told that hearing aids could make sounds <u>louder</u>

(like turning up the volume on a radio), but would not necessarily make sounds <u>clearer</u>. This thinking was reinforced by reports of unfavorable results from those hard of hearing patients who did try hearing aids and who still couldn't understand speech clearly— particularly in noisy places. Of course, it's now recognized that early attempts to fit hearing aids on people with nerve damage (sensorineural hearing loss) were seriously hindered by the limited sound quality produced by these early devices, by the limited choice of electronic variations, and by inadequate fitting strategies used in trying to determine the best manner to amplify speech without making it too loud or too noisy.

In the early days of fitting hearing aids, professionals often tried to determine who was a candidate on the basis of the degree of hearing loss shown on the hearing test. Simply considering the degree of hearing loss, however, isn't adequate to describe the impact hearing loss has on your life. Indeed, it oversimplifies the complexities of hearing impairment. By using a more "holistic" approach to identifying and correcting communication difficulties, not just hearing loss, we realize that candidacy is based more on your own personal *subjective* communicative <u>needs</u> rather than purely on test results obtained in a soundproof room. A good litmus test is to ask yourself whether you feel stressed or fatigued after a day of straining to hear. Hearing aids may simply relieve this strain, rather than making sounds louder or allowing you to understand all speech in all listening environments. Reducing strain alone can be very important, not only to you, but to those trying to talk with you. Therefore, *properly fitted hearing aids can provide benefit even if you have a very mild hearing loss.*

It was also incorrectly believed that you couldn't use hearing aids if you had normal hearing for low-pitch sounds (up to 1500 or 2000 Hz), if you had a hearing loss in only one ear, if your speech understanding abilities were reduced, or if you had difficulty tolerating loud sounds (like a crying baby). Advances in technology now allow for good fittings for most patients experiencing these problems.

Occupational and social demands vary greatly among individuals. A judge who has a mild hearing loss may desperately need amplification, while a retired person living alone with the exact same degree of hearing loss may not. You must unselfishly examine whether you're becoming a burden to others, even if you do not personally recognize difficulty hearing. *Remember that wearing hearing aids may be a symbol of courtesy to others.*

Unfortunately, despite need, many people resist trying hearing aids. There are three main reasons for this resistance.

First is *hearsay*. A lot of us have friends or relatives who have purchased hearing aids that currently reside in their dresser drawers. These unsuccessful wearers of amplification are more than happy to spread the gospel on the limitations (some accurate, some not) of hearing aids. Often, unsuccessful experiences occurred in extremely difficult listening environments in which even people with normal hearing had trouble understanding speech. Another reason some people have been unsuccessful with hearing aids is because of unrealistic expectations, and in some cases, cognitive limitations that have nothing to do with hearing itself.

Second, despite the fact that people of all ages have hearing impairment and use amplification, there has been an undeniable *social stigma* attached to wearing hearing aids. The problem of vanity has been eased, in large part, by the continuing trend toward hearing devices that can barely be seen. In fact, now, nearly all listeners with hearing loss are candidates for these very inconspicuous devices.

The third reason is the perception that the relatively high cost of hearing aids is not reflected in the value and benefits they provide. This may be a valid concern, so when making a decision as to whether this is the right time for you to try hearing aids, you must weigh whether the financial investment can be offset by the improvement in your quality of life by reducing your hearing difficulty. Be sure to consider improvements from a social, emotional, and occupational perspective, and remember to consider activities you'd like to undertake, but have given up because of communication difficulties. This is addressed in other chapters in this book.

A poorly motivated person isn't the best candidate for amplification regardless of the degree of hearing loss. From this perspective, the answer to the question of whether a steadfastly reluctant person should be forced into trying a hearing aid is probably *no*. If you're absolutely opposed to trying hearing aids at this time, and if you're convinced you'll fail, it may be advisable to wait until a later time when you are more optimistic about the process. On the other hand, keep in mind that it's <u>very possible</u> you'll be pleasantly surprised, particularly if you have realistic expectations of what hearing aids can and cannot do for you. Also, remember that, as will be discussed later in this chapter, there have been more changes in hearing aids during the last few years than in the previous forty.

"How do hearing aids work?"

Until the mid-1990s, hearing aids contained four or five basic components. Sound would enter the hearing aid through a tiny <u>microphone</u>. This sound was then converted to an electrical current that was fed into an <u>amplifier</u> and filtered by electrical components that established how much relative amplification would be provided for the different frequencies. For example, most hearing aids try to amplify the high pitches more than the low pitches. The overall amount of amplification, for most, but not all, hearing aids was then regulated by a <u>volume control</u>. The newly formed amplified electrical signal was then sent to a loudspeaker, also called a <u>receiver</u>. The receiver converted the electrical signal back into sound waves that exited the hearing aid and entered the ear canal through an earpiece or <u>earmold</u> for Behind-The-Ear (BTE) hearing aids, or through a tube located inside the plastic shell for In-The-Ear (ITE) styles. Also, all hearing aids were run by a tiny <u>battery</u>, that generally lasted for between one to three weeks. The amplification of sound just described was done using analog hearing aids. In 1996, however, the quality of amplified sound changed significantly with the introduction of the first generation of digital hearing aids.

"Are digital hearing aids better than analog hearing aids?"

A digital hearing aid has a computer chip performing the signal processing and amplification steps instead of the traditional analog circuitry described above. Digital hearing aids analyze incoming sound and convert it to a digital signal. The signal is then manipulated according to the individual's hearing levels and listening needs, reconverted to an analog form (sound waves) and delivered to the ears. It's actually a miniature computer in itself. Many of these devices produce millions of calculations per second! This was a major breakthrough in technology because it greatly increases the amount of sound processing possible in a limited amount of space. Digital hearing aids tend to have minimal distortion, advanced feedback control, improved noise suppression, and better control over directionality. They have the ability to analyze the sound environment and adapt amplification accordingly, typically making speech clearer. They also can recognize the difference between the human voice versus incoming noise to further improve speech perception. This is all done automatically without the need for volume controls. They also can wirelessly connect to many current electronic devices, such as cell phones. In addition, they allow for greater flexibility for the professional to program. We will talk about each of these features later.

"What hearing aid styles are appropriate for me?"

In the early 1950s, you would have been limited to a choice of two styles of hearing instruments: body-borne or in-eyeglass frames. These devices are almost never seen today. Now, you have many options regarding hearing aid styles (Figure 5-1).

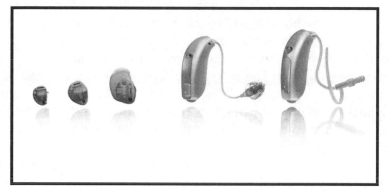

Figure 5-1: illustration of modern hearing aid styles (left to right): CIC; ITC; full shell ITE; BTE with thin wire receiver-in-canal (RIC) with stock dome; and BTE with thin tubing ready for stock earmold or dome

BTE hearing aids sit over the outer ear and are connected to an earmold located in the concha (bowl) of the ear and ear canal. BTE aids come in a variety of sizes. There are a number of options regarding the earpiece that directs sound into the ear (Figure 5-2).

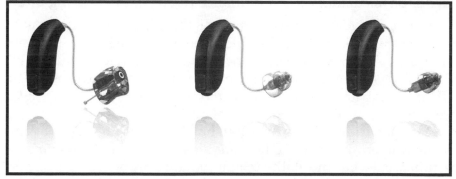

Figure 5-2: illustration of BTE hearing aids fit to custom earmold (left), instant-fit closed dome (middle), and instant fit open dome (right)

Some earmolds completely fill the ear canal while others allow for air (and sound) to get directly into the ear canal without being amplified. These devices are called *open fit* hearing aids. They first came onto the market in 2004 and have become extremely popular since they're comfortable, barely visible (unless you have no hair), and can often be fit immediately because, unlike custom hearing aids, they may not require an earmold specifically molded to your ear. Rather, they use soft domes.

Prior to 2006, nearly all BTE hearing aids sent the amplified acoustical sound through a clear plastic tube that connected the loudspeaker of the hearing aid to the earmold or dome. A more recent addition to the family of BTE styles connects the BTE style hearing aid to the receiver with a clear wire that transmits a digital (electrical) signal from the hearing aid directly to the receiver that sits inside of the ear canal. This Receiver-In-Canal (RIC) style has the advantages of eliminating unwanted resonances from the plastic tubing (that can reduce sound quality), as well as allowing for smaller instruments because the receiver is no longer housed within the part of the BTE device that sits atop your ear. The other common style of hearing aids is the custom in-the-ear (ITE). These devices include the full shell, that completely fills the bowl and ear canal, the thinner low profile, the partially occluding half concha, the in-the-canal (ITC), and the tiniest of ITE hearing aids, the completely-in-canal (CIC).

While cosmetic considerations may be important, the decision as to which style hearing aid is most appropriate for you should be based on both <u>physical</u> as well as <u>audiological</u> factors.

"What physical factors can influence fitting of my hearing aids?"

Anatomical characteristics may dictate the style; for example, BTE hearing aids may not be able to be used if you have deformed outer ears. The depth of your concha may determine the suitability of ITE model instruments, and in order to be able to wear the ITC or CIC type instruments, your ear canal must not be so curvy that it prevents easy insertion and removal.

Manual dexterity is important in handling hearing aids. Not only is removal and insertion of hearing aids somewhat challenging for certain people, but the ability to manipulate controls and the battery must be considered and assessed before you decide that a certain style is right for you. Always ask your hearing professional to show you the different styles, and if possible, to let you handle and try these devices prior to purchasing. Keep in mind, however, that learning to insert or remove the hearing aid from your ear, or the battery from the hearing aid, may take a little practice, so don't get discouraged if you can't do it the first time you try.

Some people need hearing aids or earmolds that are large enough to accommodate a <u>vent</u> (hole) drilled into it, so that air can enter your ear canal. Without this *ventilation*, you may perceive a "plugged up" feeling or you may sound to yourself like you're in a barrel when you speak. This phenomenon is called the "occlusion effect." You can demonstrate this to yourself by sticking your finger in your ear and counting out loud. People who have similar hearing in each ear and who have nerve damage will find that their own voice shifts toward the blocked ear. This happens because when we vocalize, our ear canal vibrates and this vibration leaks out of the ear and into the air without being noticed. But when you block your ear, as some hearing aids, earmolds or domes do, the vibration gets trapped in your ear canal and you may hear an echo or sound like you're talking from inside a barrel. Some people find CIC hearing aids are particularly prone to this occlusion effect. Also, for some, CIC hearing aids can be uncomfortable because they may extend deeply into the ear canal and may be physically uncomfortable because the skin is much thinner in the inner part of the canal than it is at the outer portion.

Some styles of hearing aid, particularly the open fit BTE devices that are attached to non-occluding open earpieces (those that don't block your ear canals) may be more comfortable to wear and don't create this occlusion effect. In addition, if your ears produce excessive cerumen (earwax), are very hairy or prone to excessive sweating, you may be better off with BTE rather than ITE devices. Fortunately, wax guards are now available for most hearing aids so the number of repair needs due to wax blocking the receiver of the hearing aids have been greatly reduced. And, certain hearing aids are more resistant to water and sweat than others.

Medical contraindications such as draining ears or other medical problems may prevent the use of any hearing aid apparatus blocking your ear canals. In this instance, you'll need open, non-occluding earmolds or possibly bone conduction-type systems. These types of hearing aids are beyond the scope of this discussion, but can be reviewed by your hearing healthcare provider if applicable to you.

"What audiological factors will influence my fitting?"

The *audiometric pattern* on your audiogram may show certain frequencies (pitches) that have normal hearing. For example, if you have a high frequency hearing loss, but have normal hearing in low frequencies, you may be best served by non-occluding systems to allow low-pitched sounds to pass into your ear without being amplified. Conversely, if you have a hearing loss in low frequencies, it's necessary to keep low frequency amplification in your ear, so a hearing aid that fills the ear canal may be necessary.

The *degree of loss* may dictate the need for a specific kind of hearing aid. For example, profound hearing losses are best served by BTE-style hearing aids with closed earmolds. Milder losses, however, can be fit with almost any style of hearing aid.

Special features may be important for you, such as directional microphones (that primarily amplify signals coming from in front of you and will be discussed later) and/or the addition of a telecoil (a magnetic induction loop). Telecoils allow sound to bypass the hearing aid microphone and amplify signals received electromagnetically (eg., from telephones). In addition to allowing you to listen on the telephone without feedback (whistling), telecoils can interface with a variety of assistive listening devices (see Appendix I). CIC hearing aids are generally too small to contain these special, and often much needed, components.

Conversely, a potential advantage of CIC hearing aids is that the microphone lies either within, or at the entrance of the ear canal and thus is able to benefit fully from the *natural amplification* of the outer ear and concha bowl. The receiver of the hearing aid is also frequently located closer to the eardrum, where the amount of air trapped in the ear canal that needs to vibrate is less than for most other fittings. Therefore, *less hearing aid amplification may be needed* to produce the same sound pressure at the eardrum. Reducing the amount of amplification a hearing aid provides potentially results in lower distortion levels and less likelihood of acoustic feedback.

Acoustic feedback refers to the whistling or buzzing sound often produced when you cup your hand or hold a telephone over your ear while wearing a hearing aid. It also occurs when the hearing aid or earmold is not properly or snugly inserted in your ear. It happens because the sound amplified by the hearing aid leaks out of your ear canal and goes back into the microphone of the hearing aid where it is re-amplified. Feedback from hearing aids can be annoying not only to you, but to others. It's not acceptable, except momentarily when covering your ear or inserting the device into your ear. The more amplification required (because of your degree of hearing loss), the more likely it is that feedback could occur. Generally speaking, the closer the microphone where the sound enters) is to the exit point of the amplified sound from the hearing aid or earmold, the greater the likelihood of feedback. BTE hearing aids, therefore, often have an advantage over ITC or CIC styles since there's more physical distance between the microphone and the receiver. However, if you use an open fit BTE that doesn't block your ear, there is an even larger opening through which amplified sound can leak back into the microphone. Fortunately, most digital hearing aids (of all styles) now contain "active feedback management" systems. An active system detects feedback and counteracts it before it occurs by creating mirror-image cancelling signals or predetermining the feedback pathway, thus, eliminating or at least minimizing the feedback.

Even with digital feedback control, it's still important that earmolds, domes, or hearing aid shells fit properly in your ears for both comfort and retention. This is why it's essential that your hearing healthcare professional takes good impressions of your ears before you obtain custom fit hearing aids. If you've never had an earmold impression taken, don't worry. It doesn't hurt. Your provider will first place a cotton or foam block in your ear canal and then inject viscous material in your ear that will harden in about five minutes. It's a similar process to getting impressions made by the dentist, except thankfully, you don't need a Novocaine shot! And recently, some professionals have begun using a 3D scanning technique that takes an image of your ear canal without even having to make an impression.

Some hearing impaired listeners have no usable hearing for very high frequencies. Thus, no matter how much amplification the hearing aid provides for those sounds, the damaged ear simply can't handle them without perceiving distortion. Certain hearing aids contain a feature called *frequency lowering* in which the unusable high frequency sounds are actually shifted down to a lower frequency that the ear can properly use.

It's not unusual to find that the most important factors determining success or failure of a fitting are those unrelated to audiometric findings. For example, all of the following have to be taken into consideration: your age; your general physical and mental health; your motivation (as opposed to that of your family's); your finances; your cosmetic preferences; and your communication needs. It's heartening to note that the primary reasons for rejection of hearing aids, after people try them, are less related to finances and cosmetics, and more to do with difficulty hearing in background noise, and discomfort from loud sounds. These problems, while still not completely gone, have been greatly lessened by modern-day hearing aids and fitting techniques.

"How do I adjust the volume so that I can hear soft sounds, yet loud sounds don't overwhelm me?"

A lot of people don't realize that when you have a hearing loss due to nerve damage (sensorineural), your hearing problem is primarily limited to difficulty hearing soft sounds. Your ability to hear loud sounds may be okay. In fact, many people with sensorineural hearing loss find louder sounds to be uncomfortable. So, there are three basic rules that must be followed if a hearing aid fitting is to be successful:

1. soft sounds must be made audible (so that you can hear them);
2. normal conversational sounds must be comfortable; and
3. loud sounds must not be uncomfortable.

The way to achieve this goal is with a technology called *compression*. In the past, hearing aids would provide the same amount of amplification to soft incoming sounds as they would for loud incoming sounds. The technical term for this is *linear* amplification. This would allow people to hear soft sounds, but loud sounds would then be uncomfortable or even painful. Many wearers reported that in order to hear soft sounds, they had to turn their hearing aids up too high. This did indeed allow them to hear soft sounds, but it also produced the undesirable effect of making loud sounds uncomfortable. Imagine a certain level of sound enters the hearing aid, let's say 65 dB (that happens to be about the level of normal conversational speech). To make this speech comfortable, the volume of the hearing aid might be set so that it produces 25 dB of amplification. Therefore, 90 dB comes into the ear canal (65 plus 25). Now, imagine that the sound coming into the hearing aid suddenly becomes much louder, as might occur in a restaurant when people at your table start to laugh at a joke. If you're wearing a linear aid, the sound coming into it is now increased to 80 dB, and this type of hearing aid will still add 25 dB of amplification, so the sound in your ear canal increases to 105 dB. For most people, this will be entirely too loud and uncomfortable, and your reaction will be to try and turn it down using the volume control. This is why you might have seen people with linear hearing aids adjusting the volume control quite often when sound intensity in the surrounding environment changed.

In 1992, a new type of hearing aid was introduced using more advanced technology called *non-linear*, or *dynamic range compression*. With this, there's more amplification given to soft sounds than there is for louder sounds. In other words, when sounds are above a certain level set in the hearing aid, it's as if an invisible finger reaches up and automatically moves the volume down for you, and vice versa, when the sound environment becomes lower than a certain level it moves the volume up for you.

This type of non-linear hearing aid basically squeezes a wide range of loudness into a narrower range, which has generated the other descriptive name of *compression hearing aids*. Going back to the earlier example, now with the non-linear type, when sounds entering the hearing aid suddenly increase to 80 dB, the amplification may be automatically lowered from 25 dB to 10 dB. Therefore, the sound reaching your eardrum is a more comfortable.

There were two big problems with this early form of compression. The first was that when loud sounds would enter the hearing aid microphone, it would trigger a change in amplification such that *all* sounds were reduced to maintain comfort. This was called *single channel compression*. The problem with this is that an individual's loudness growth pattern may be different from one pitch to another. That is, you might find that high-pitched sounds (like dishes clanging) seem painfully loud to you but low-pitched sounds (a refrigerator humming) do not. Therefore, the amount of compression needed to be different for various frequencies. This is where the next step up in the evolution of compression comes in, *non-linear multiple channel compression*. Hearing aids with multiple channels can divide the incoming signal into as few as three, or as many as over twenty channels.

With multiple channel compression, characteristics of the hearing aid will be tailored to your personal needs based upon how loud you interpret certain sounds to be for various frequencies. Perhaps there will be a lot of compression for the high frequencies but very little for the low frequencies. Compression helps to make sounds appear comfortably loud for you.

The second thing multichannel compression accomplishes may be even more important. If your hearing aid system has only one channel, a loud noise made up of mostly low frequencies (as might be found in cocktail parties) would instruct the hearing aid that it needs to lower its amplification for all frequencies. This would help to keep the sound from being too loud, but it would make some of the high frequency sounds (like consonants) too soft to hear. On the other hand, a multichannel hearing aid, in that same loud low frequency noise situation, would decrease the amplification for low frequencies, making sound comfortable without changing the amplification for the high frequencies (thus preserving audibility of important high frequency consonant sounds). This system can actually produce additional high frequency amplification while simultaneously reducing low frequency amplification, all depending on the sound environment.

Non-linear, multiple channel hearing aids act not only as a means of loudness control, but also as a means of differentiating the amount of amplification given to different parts of the speech signal. If fitted correctly, they can dampen the strong elements of speech, such as vowels, and enhance the delicate speech elements such as the /s/, /sh/ and /f/ sounds. This can improve speech clarity, especially in difficult listening environments. In addition, as discussed below, multi-channel compression plays an important role in minimizing the adverse effects of background noise. This will be explained in the next section.

Hearing aids containing multichannel compression can regulate themselves so automatically that they frequently don't contain a volume control. You may find this to your liking if you're the type who doesn't like to frequently adjust your hearing aids, or, you may feel that not having a volume control takes away too much control from you. This is something you should discuss carefully with your hearing healthcare provider.

"Will my hearing aids help me when I'm in background noise?"

We live in a noisy world. Many people with hearing loss correctly believe that they can hear pretty well in quiet, but as soon as there's background noise, like in a restaurant or a room with lots of people talking, their understanding is poor. The truth is, people with hearing loss typically have more trouble understanding speech in noise even if they can hear the speech than do people with normal hearing. Hearing aids in the past were not very good at separating speech from noise. The strategy was that if the hearing aid reduced the amplification for the low frequencies, where typically there was a lot of noise energy, you would be able to hear speech better. The problem was that while this approach might indeed reduce the loudness of the noise, it also tended to make speech softer and the sound quality less desirable. This occurred since speech has a lot of the same, primarily low frequency (pitch) sound energy as noise. As digital processing became more sophisticated, newer and better methods of controlling noise have emerged. One of these approaches, called *noise reduction*, works on a different principle. Even though speech and noise can have similar energy in terms of pitch, the temporal (timing) and the amplitude (loudness) characteristics of the signals are quite different. The computerized processing contained in certain hearing aids can measure and calculate these characteristics and thus estimate what is speech and what is noise. Then, similar to the way multiple channel compression works, the digital processor can limit the amount of amplification for those channels (bands) that are judged to contain more noise than speech, or conversely, provide full amplification in the bands that contain more speech than noise. Noise reduction doesn't necessarily make speech clearer when it is immersed in a lot of background noise, but it can make the background seem much more comfortable, while multichannel compression actually can help enhance speech understanding by reducing the amplification in the channels that contain the most noise, and increasing the amplification in the channels than contain the most speech.

Another approach to controlling noise also can make speech in noise clearer. Typically, you face the person who is speaking to you. Noise, however, may originate in front, behind, and/or to your sides. Many hearing aids now contain *directional* or *multiple microphones* that "communicate" with each other so that sounds originating from the front of the hearing aid receive maximum amplification, and sounds originating from the sides or behind receive less amplification. This effectively suppresses some (though not all) of the annoying background noise that may create so much difficulty for you. When you wear hearing aids with multiple or directional microphones, you can try to position yourself in a room so that noise is less bothersome. For example, in a restaurant, you should take a seat that has you facing out with your back toward the center of the room where most of the noise is located, or similarly, away from the kitchen.

Of course, if you're a taxi driver, or if you need to hear children in the back seat when you're driving, you may be better off with hearing aids that amplify sounds equally from all directions. Another example of when you might want amplification to occur from all around you would be when listening to music. Some hearing aids allow you to select whether you want most of the amplification to occur for signals in front of you or whether you want equal amplification for signals all around you. Some hearing aids will allow you to touch a button on the hearing aid or in a remote control that will turn on the directional function, while even more automatically turn on this function automatically whenever it detects noise. Another exciting new feature of digital hearing aids with directional or multiple microphones is that the directional function can be adaptive. This means that not only will the hearing aid automatically switch into the directional mode, but it will determine exactly where the noise is coming from and specifically target those directions for a reduction in amplification. This adaptive directionality can be especially useful considering the fact that the location of unwanted noise is not always directly behind you and is certainly not always coming from the same direction.

It's also important to know that multiple microphones require a minimal space requirement of at least 3mm between the microphones. Because of their small size, CIC hearing aids are unable to accommodate this useful feature, though some natural directivity is achieved by the placement of CICs within the ear canal.

No hearing aids effectively eliminate all background noise. If all the sound energy that makes up noise were eliminated, important segments of speech also would be missing, and remember that normal listeners also experience background noise daily. If all background noise were eliminated, the acoustic world would be quite boring and unnatural. Even so, don't hesitate to discuss your experience with background noise with your provider so that your hearing aids can be fine-tuned to reach the best compromise. Thus, we must face the reality that some environments are simply too noisy for hard of hearing <u>or</u> normal hearing people to comfortably converse. In those situations, no matter how good the hearing aids are, you may still have problems.

"I like to listen to music. Can hearing aids help?"

Hearing aids are certainly able to make musical sounds audible (capable of being heard) that you might not hear without amplification. However, if some of the same strategies that are applied to listening to speech were applied to listening to music, there might be some problems. For example, while noise reduction can be helpful for reducing unpleasant noise, your hearing aids could be "tricked" into believing that certain parts of music are noise, and they would then reduce the amplification for those parts of the music. Of course, one might argue that some of the music that is heard these days really is nothing more than noise, but that is another story! So programs designed for music should not employ noise reduction. In addition, as mentioned earlier, part of the enjoyment of music is having the sounds enter each ear from a variety of directions. So here again, while multiple and directional microphones are really helpful when listening to speech, you're better off listening to music with hearing aids that amplify equally from all directions. Fortunately, most of the new hearing aids that contain the directional feature, will allow you to either turn off this feature manually or will automatically do so for you. Another difference in the strategies used in hearing music as opposed to speech is that music programs don't use so much compression. The reason for this is so that the full range of musical sounds (from soft to loud) is preserved.

Another limitation in hearing aids, relative to home stereo systems, is that the *bandwidth* (number of frequencies amplified by the hearing aid) is more restricted. While the bandwidth of hearing aids keeps getting wider, there are presently some limits because of the very small loudspeaker (receiver) that is contained in hearing aids and the fact that hearing aids are powered by a battery that provides only a small amount of current (compared to plugging your home stereo into a wall outlet).

"How do hearing aids know which features and which programs to use?"

Once you and your hearing care provider have selected the appropriate hearing aids and features based on your communication needs, the devices may be programmed to contain multiple programs (typically two to four), that are specifically designed for different situations, such as listening in quiet, listening in noise, adjusting for comfort in constant noise (like in your car), listening to music, or listening to the telephone. You can select which program is best for different situations by pressing a button on the hearing aid or remote control. Alternatively, you may choose to have the hearing aid work in an *automatic mode* in which it makes selection of the optimal program based on characteristics of sounds entering the hearing aid. Multiple programs can also be very useful if you have a fluctuating hearing loss such as in Ménière's disease.

"Will I be able to hear on my cell phone?"

It's very important that you're able to use the telephone with your hearing aids. Too frequently, hearing aid users believe they must remove their hearing aids when they talk on the phone because otherwise they get feedback. Not only is this annoying and embarrassing, but it makes hearing the voice at the other end of the call especially hard. To combat this problem, BTE and ITE (but not CIC) hearing aids can contain a *telecoil*, a small metal inductance coil hidden within the aid that picks up and amplifies electro-magnetic leakage produced from telephones and in doing so, creates a magnetic loop through which the desired signal passes. When the telecoil is activated, you have the option to turn off the microphone to eliminate feedback or undesirable environmental sounds. Telecoils also are used to interface with various assistive listening devices (as discussed in Chapter 12 and Appendix I). To activate the telecoil program, you can either press a button on the aid, use a remote control, or get a hearing aid that automatically switches itself into the telecoil mode as soon as it detects electromagnetic leakage from the phone. Then, when you remove the phone from your ear, the hearing aid automatically switches back into the normal listening program.

Certain cellular phones can create a buzzing static or interference if used with a hearing aid telecoil and are therefore incompatible with telecoil usage. However, FCC regulations have forced wireless phone manufacturers to not only produce more cell phone models that will work with hearing aids, but also to provide a numerical rating for their cell phone efficiency. It's a very good idea to find out if your hearing aid will work with a cell phone before you buy a new phone and before you purchase hearing aids. The best way to do this is to try it out first.

For hearing aids that don't contain telecoils, such as CICs (that are too small to house the inductance coil), the use of multiple programs can be effective by dedicating one program to a frequency response that de-emphasizes amplification in the high frequencies where feedback might be produced. This works because most telephones don't transduce sounds in very high frequencies anyway.

Be sure to tell your hearing care professional what kind of a telephone system you use. For example, if you use a Bluetooth telephone, some hearing aids can offer you a feature that will wirelessly interface your hearing aids to the Bluetooth phone. This is a very nice wireless hands-free feature that could actually allow you to hear the telephone in both ears. In fact, many hearing aids now have wireless communication between binaural hearing aids. This can be very helpful so that when automatic changes occur in one hearing aid, the other one can also adapt in order to preserve important acoustic information. And speaking of binaural listening, you could even wirelessly listen through your hearing aids to music downloaded onto your phone or iPod or MP3 player.

"If my hearing changes are my hearing aids obsolete?"

Don't worry. Most digital hearing aids have sufficient programming flexibility that will allow your hearing professional to adjust your hearing aids to a wide range to account for most audiometric configurations, while also allowing for adjustment for your individual loudness comfort levels. Of course, there are some limitations. Hearing aids appropriate for a mild or moderate degree of hearing loss won't be powerful enough for someone with a profound loss. Similarly, the style of the hearing aid may limit the fitting range. For instance, you can't use open fit devices if you suddenly develop a substantial loss in low frequencies.

"How will I know if I'm properly using hearing aids and if they're properly programmed?"

A feature available in some hearing aids is referred to as *datalogging*. This feature can provide your professional with information about the number of hours you wear the hearing aids, the relative amount of time you spend in each program, how often you change the controls, and even the percentage of time you spend in different acoustic environments. Some hearing aids are even considered "trainable" because they'll automatically adjust their programming based on the information obtained from the datalog. This datalogging information can be quite informative to both you and to the professional who programs your hearing aids to meet your needs.

"Is there ever going to be a disposable hearing aid?"

There have been some attempts in the past to manufacture disposable and entry-level hearing aids. A potential advantage of these devices is that your initial investment may be less and the devices may not be as susceptible to technological obsolescence because they're designed for temporary use. Thus, after a limited period of time, if you decide that the hearing aids aren't meeting your needs, they can be discarded and no further money is invested, kind of like disposable contact lenses. To date, however, none have achieved widespread acceptance due to physical comfort and ethical concerns regarding the methods with which they're dispensed to the public. Recently however, one manufacturer introduced a new device that fits halfway down the ear canal and is completely invisible. The device is designed to be worn 24 hours a day, and it lasts for up to three months. When the instrument battery expires the entire aid is discarded and replaced with a new one by a trained hearing professional who has access to a microscope for safe insertion into the ear canal. The hearing aid is sold on an annual subscription basis. Thus in the long run, it may be more expensive than a hearing aid designed to last for 3-5 years. There are some restrictions on who can use this device. You must have healthy ear canals that are of the correct diameter, shape, depth, and free of bony obstructions, skin conditions or frequent and excessive earwax accumulation.

"What limitations might I expect with hearing aids?"

Hearing aids are meant to improve ease of communication and minimize listening fatigue. They're not meant to allow you to "hear a pin drop," and there are going to be circumstances in which hearing aids don't give you all the benefits you'd like. The most frequent complaints voiced by some hearing aid wearers are that some sounds become too loud to bear and some speech remains unclear.

With regard to clarity, remember that hearing aids are <u>aides</u> to hearing. They're not new ears, and they cannot correct for certain limitations in understanding that are more related to severe inner ear distortion, decline in cognition, and poor listening habits. If the hearing aid wearer has cognitive deficits, such as senility or Alzheimer's, the hearing aids may not provide maximum communication ability, no matter how well the instruments may be functioning.

Another common limitation of hearing aids is that you may have more difficulty hearing when the sound source is at a distance from you. This occurs, for example, in large conference rooms or auditoriums. Loudness (intensity) decreases as physical distance increases. Unfortunately, most background noise surrounds you, so while the intensity of speech decreases with distance, the intensity of noise may not. This is one reason why hearing aids effectively transmit sound if a person talks right into the microphone, but at longer, more realistic distances, reception diminishes. It would be ideal if sound produced at the source transferred directly to you without losing any intensity. It's obviously impractical, however, to ask someone speaking to you to constantly move closer to your ear.

One way to achieve this effect is with *direct audio input*, where the person speaking holds or wears a microphone. Unfortunately, many hearing aid wearers are reluctant to ask others to use a microphone or wear a wired device. Direct audio input also allows you to plug in a remote microphone or an FM assistive listening system, connect directly to a TV, or connect to other devices such as your computer, MP3, iPod, radio, and so forth (see Chapter Twelve and Appendix I).

An alternative approach is to use instruments called assistive listening devices that transmit by wireless FM (like a radio), infrared, or induction loop. You may have seen these devices in auditoriums and theaters, and they can be used in combination with your hearing aids. Ask your hearing care professional if the particular hearing aids you're considering will be able to work with these extra features.

"What should I expect with my new hearing aids?"

Hearing aids are electronic devices and sometimes not perfect. Since the main goal of amplification is to help communication, recognize that it may take some time to fully adjust to your new hearing. Don't be disappointed if you experience only minimal benefit during the initial trial with amplification. Talk with your hearing professional to determine what you should and shouldn't expect to be able to do when you begin your new life with hearing aids.

The benefit derived from amplification may be subtle. If your new hearing aids ease your daily listening tasks, they're beneficial. Depending on your hearing loss, the goal of hearing aids may not be to make sounds louder. That is, especially where only high frequency amplification occurs, there are only a few English language sounds in this range (such as /s/, /sh/, /t/, /th/, /f/ and /k/). Therefore, your high frequency hearing aids are designed to pick up only these consonants and since we're talking about relatively few sounds, the benefits of amplification may not be readily apparent. It's important to note here that even though we're speaking of a few sounds, these sounds are critically important.

You also need to recognize that prediction of guaranteed long-term benefit from amplification is difficult to determine. A period of initial adjustment and a learning process is required for most new hearing aid users. It may take several weeks before you adjust to the new pattern of sound and learn new "recognition" cues that you probably have not heard for a long time. As a new wearer, you need to be oriented to the world of amplification. You may require a gradual "break-in" wearing schedule (a few hours the first day, six hours the second, nine hours the third, etc.), or you may be encouraged to wear the hearing aids immediately during all your waking hours. You may require additional counseling and training, either individually or in groups with others with hearing loss, and family members.

You must accept that time is required for adapting to hearing aids. At first, your brain may interpret the new sounds you are hearing as being too loud or too prevalent. Even though it's likely that your brain will adapt to these newly heard signals, you can get hearing aids that contain an *acclimatization* feature. With this feature the amount of amplification will initially be reduced, but the hearing aid can be programmed to gradually increase the amplification automatically at intervals agreed upon by you and your hearing healthcare professional.

Your ability to understand amplified speech can continue to grow for as long as three months following the use of new hearing aids. Most professionals will give you a one-month trial period with new hearing aids. If market conditions allow, trial periods may be extended. My advice is, if a trial period is not offered, take your business elsewhere!

It's important that you read the instruction manual that comes with your hearing aids. Hopefully, your provider will have told you everything you need to know about inserting and removing your hearing aids, checking the batteries, cleaning and maintaining the instruments, and using hearing aids with the telephone. But often, too much information can overload the brain. Take the hearing aids home, read the instruction manual (or check out the information on the manufacturer's website), and don't be afraid to call your provider if you have any questions. Then go out and wear them in a variety of listening environments. When you return to your hearing healthcare provider for follow-up visits, discuss the situations with which you may have had difficulty so that possible adjustments and fine-tuning can be achieved.

Also remember that hearing aids are sophisticated electronic devices that spend most of their time in a rather unfriendly environment—your ear. Can you imagine what would happen if you placed your home stereo system in a rainforest? Well, your ear canal is somewhat like a rainforest in that it is very warm (about 98.6 degrees), it's moist (with earwax), and it doesn't always receive enough fresh air. As such, hearing aids do require occasional repair. As mentioned earlier, blockage from earwax, even though greatly minimized by the use of small "wax traps" can still occur. You can minimize the need for repair if you're conscientious about cleaning your hearing aids daily according to instructions, ensuring that the wax traps are not blocked, and possibly storing the hearing aids every night in a dehumidifier that soaks up any excess moisture.

Last, but certainly not least, recognize that hearing is not the same as listening. Hearing simply refers to the audibility of sounds. The purpose of your hearing aids is to provide you with access to the comfortable sounds you've been missing. But listening requires your attention and focus. I'll bet you know of friends (or possibly family members) who have normal hearing, but are very bad listeners (see Chapter Three, Q&A#7). Supplementing your new hearing aids with additional rehabilitation methods such as home-based auditory training, group therapy, speechreading lessons, assistive listening devices, and so forth, can be very useful in giving you the kinds of communication strategies that can make the difference between understanding and being left out of a conversation, particularly in tough listening environments. Talk to your professional about establishing a comprehensive communication enhancement plan for you.

Conclusions

Now you have the facts, at least as they stand today. Remember, in order to have the best chance of succeeding with hearing aids, be patient with yourself, have a sense of humor, and maintain realistic expectations. You and your brain have consciously and subconsciously created many behaviors over the years to compensate for your hearing loss. Some of the habits you've picked up have probably helped your ability to communicate, but some may have actually impaired your communication skills. Properly fit hearing aids can give you back some of those sounds you've been missing, but you have to learn how to properly use your hearing aids and supplement your new hearing with better listening habits. Don't hesitate to contact your hearing professional when you have any questions. It's not easy to master all the new features available in hearing aids, so ask for instruction and inform your provider about the aspects of your communication that you're happy with as well as those you still wish to improve.

CHAPTER SIX
Fitness and Better Hearing
Helaine M. Alessio, PhD
Kathleen Hutchinson Marron, PhD

Dr. Alessio is a Professor and Chair of the Department of Kinesiology and Health at Miami University (Oxford, OH). She uses animal and human models to investigate benefits and risks of exercise and sedentary lifestyles. With colleague Kathy Hutchinson-Marron, she has investigated the role of cardiovascular health and fitness in influencing hearing acuity in people of all ages, fitness levels and noise exposures. Together, they have published many research papers that have been widely cited. She has also studied physiological parameters associated with exercise-induced oxidative stress. Her research has been supported by the National Cancer Institute, National Institutes of Health, and National Institute on Aging.

Dr. Hutchinson Marron is Chair of the Department of Speech Pathology and Audiology and is on the executive board of the Center for Disability Studies. She is a Professor and faculty associate of the Center for Human Development, Teaching and Learning (Miami University). Her research interests include study of the relation of fitness and muscle strength to hearing and susceptibility to hearing loss. Her research also focuses on meta-analysis techniques to study cross-cultural perceptions of individuals with craniofacial disorders, techniques to evaluate auditory processing disorders, and evoked potential responses among athletes with concussions. She teaches clinical courses in audiology, research methodology and courses in disability studies.

Noise exposure and age seem to be two main culprits associated with hearing loss. Given enough time and exposure to noise either at work, leisure or short-term exposure to very loud noise (such as from firearms or loud music), hearing acuity is likely to decline with age. However, recent evidence has accumulated identifying factors that have little to do with age or noise exposure, yet have a significant influence on hearing acuity. Some of these factors include marital status, education, personality type, and health and fitness.

Recent evidence has demonstrated that although aging plays a part, factors other than age impact the rate at which sensorineural hearing loss occurs. In particular, as remarkable as it may sound, cardiovascular (CV) health and fitness have been studied and found to influence hearing. CV health and fitness can be measured in a variety of ways and is often assessed in a rested and fasted state through the collection and analyses of blood for lipids. This would include cholesterol and triglyceride levels that indicate how well blood flows and delivers oxygen throughout the body. The more cholesterol and triglycerides in the blood, the more blockages there are in blood vessels. This can result in excessive stress that can damage the heart in its effort to circulate blood and oxygen throughout the body. Another measure of CV health and fitness includes a graded exercise test that utilizes either a stationary bicycle or treadmill. A person's heart rate is monitored, and breathing is analyzed for oxygen consumption, then converted to units of measure (such as maximal oxygen uptake). This is represented as VO_2max and will be used throughout this chapter. VO_2max is the maximum amount of oxygen that a person can breathe in with their lungs, pump out with their heart, and send via blood to working muscles for energy. It represents the CV system's ability to function at peak capacity and is considered a benchmark measure of CV health and fitness. Heart rate and the amount of oxygen you can get into your cells (VO_2) can be measured when biking, walking or running at increasing workloads until you can no longer continue due to fatigue, or until a preset target of intensity is reached. <u>There is overwhelming evidence that regular exercise can increase VO_2max by 10-25 percent</u>, and the higher the VO_2max, the lower the risk for heart disease, hearing loss and premature death from all causes. The overall benefit of exercise cannot be overemphasized.

Figure 6-1 (opposite page) shows the association between VO_2max and mortality (as measured by number of deaths in 10,000 persons). Individuals with VO_2max values that were in the low-fit category (below 31ml/kg/minute for women and below 34 ml/kg/minute for men, were at higher risk for metabolic and cardiovascular diseases including obesity, diabetes, and stroke. Those with VO_2max values greater than 31ml/kg/min for women and greater than 34 ml/kg/ minute for men, benefited by reducing those metabolic and cardiovascular risk factors and also having better hearing acuity.

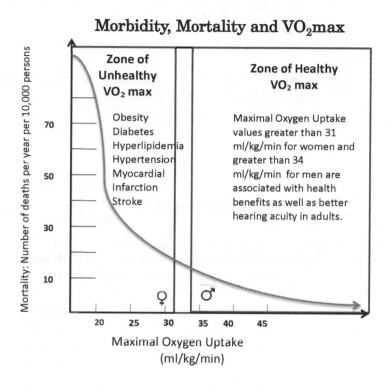

Figure 6-1: association between VO_2max and mortality

Why, When and How Should I get my Health Evaluated?

Former Secretary-General of the United Nations Kofi Annan is quoted as having said, "Knowledge is power. Information is liberating." Not knowing one's health risk status may on the one hand contribute to a stress-free state of mind. On the other hand, the reality of one's health risks eventually reveals itself, often in premature diseases that may have been avoided or mitigated with appropriate and timely intervention. A special category of diseases called "Silent Diseases" are described as those that produce minimal or no symptoms, although if left untreated may result in severe, life-changing or even fatal consequences. The number one silent disease that is also considered a *silent killer* is heart disease. Risk factors include hypertension, smoking, sedentary lifestyle, obesity and high cholesterol and triglycerides—all of which can be measured. You can start a health-promoting intervention likely to include lifestyle change, stress management, and/or in many cases pharmaceutical intervention by:

- assessing blood pressure
- quantifying the number of cigarettes smoked on a daily basis
- measuring the number of steps taken per day or time (in minutes) spent in physical activity
- measuring or predicting VO_2max
- assessing body composition
- knowing your blood lipid profile

In some cases, surgical intervention (e.g., angioplasty, gastric bypass, coronary artery bypass) is necessary, especially in cases where a silent disease is left unchecked for too long and damage has occurred in the heart or blood vessels. Those with metabolic disorders are also at risk. Once repaired, however, most patients who had a variety of CV conditions, including blocked arteries and congestive heart failure among others, can return to normal, productive lives.

So, if knowledge is power and information is liberating, then it's important that <u>assessment of cardiovascular health and hearing occur early and often</u>. How early and how often? Answers to these questions depend on many factors including the typical health and hearing screenings that occur at schools, in annual medical visits often designated as preventive or wellness visits, or at diagnostic health visits. These procedures are initiated as a result of problems perceived by individuals themselves, or by family members, friends or teachers who notice signs and symptoms of health or hearing deficits.

Typical health evaluations include an assessment of health risk based on physical, mental and social health. Regular health and wellness visits begin shortly after birth. By the time individuals reach school age, regular annual visits are expected and even required for enrollment by many school systems. After high school, annual health and wellness visits are typically done on a voluntary basis, although some occupations may require them. Tracking height, weight, body composition, blood pressure, blood lipids, blood glucose, sight, hearing, reflexes and results of a physical examination are all part of a comprehensive wellness visit. Furthermore, information about behaviors that affect health, such as smoking, medications, drugs, alcohol, stress and social support, among others, all provide valuable information about your health status and measures your health risk. These assessments are typically performed by a medical professional such as a physician, nurse or chiropractor. Some tests come and go, depending on cost and evidence-based research that supports their value and their association with life-threatening diseases. The American Heart Association recommends tests for blood pressure, blood lipids, blood glucose, height, weight and specific health behaviors (especially smoking and alcohol) be performed on individuals age 20 years and older at least every two years.

Health and hearing assessments provide knowledge about one's functional health status. This information can be useful for disease prediction. This knowledge can also serve as a powerful motivator to maintain or change certain behaviors that may range from subtle adjustments in diet, exercise or noise exposure, to more extreme interventions. One such example is the decision by celebrity Angelina Jolie in 2013 to undergo a double mastectomy when she learned she carried mutations in critical breast cancer genes. Information about one's relative risk and functional capabilities can be affirming or alarming. However, in either case it can also be liberating. Whether one agrees or disagrees with Angelina Jolie's decision, a major issue is that knowledge she received from her healthcare provider motivated her to choose a course of action to address her specific health risk. Once you have and understand information about your health and hearing status, then you're free to make choices that are appropriate for your unique situation. Inaction or inappropriate action may cause a minor health or hearing condition to unravel to a serious life quality issue or life threatening condition.

Annual CV health assessments are recommended for all healthy people and typically include assessment of:

- blood pressure
- body weight and height
- blood lipids
- a physical exam
- breast or prostate examination
- and other tests specific to a person's family and personal health risk, depending on age.

The U.S. Preventive Services Task Force did not endorse a recommendation for annual hearing screening for asymptomatic adults age 50 years and older because of lack of evidence in the balance of benefits and harm.[1] The Task Force did, however, recommend that adults age 50 and older who perceived hearing problems be assessed for objective hearing impairment and when indicated by signs and symptoms, be treated appropriately.

Exercise is Medicine for Health and Hearing

When an intervention is required to prevent further deterioration of the cardiovascular system, improve its function or assist in recovery from an invasive surgical operation, one intriguing intervention has proven particularly beneficial. This intervention has been shown to have a dose-response effect that mimics (and in some cases exceeds) the effects of traditional medicine, with little to no side effects. *The intervention is exercise!* Decades of research investigating the benefits and risks of regular exercise have provided overwhelming scientific evidence demonstrating that in most adults, the beneficial effects of exercise far outweigh any risks, including sudden death and acute injuries. Conclusions from exercise research include case studies to clinical trials, and have resulted in a general recommendation that a program of regular exercise should include cardiorespiratory, resistance, flexibility, and neuromotor exercise training beyond activities of daily living. Regular exercise is necessary to improve and maintain physical fitness and health and is essential for most adults. This knowledge is gradually moving from the scientific arena to clinical settings where personal physicians are sitting down with their patients and asking them about their exercise habits. When patients share that they are sedentary (about 25 percent are) and admit that they don't achieve a minimal amount of daily activity, physicians often recommend a course of action to change them from a couch potato to a physically active lifestyle.

Understanding the correct intensity and duration of exercise is critical to understanding the role of exercise as medicine. And exercise is medicine! A new initiate from the largest sports medicine and exercise science organization in the world (the American College of Sports Medicine—ACSM), along with the American Heart Association and the American Academy of Family Physicians is in fact called *Exercise is Medicine.*™ A goal of this campaign is to start discussions between healthcare providers and every American to ensure that exercise is front and center in every discussion on disease prevention health and wellness. The belief that exercise and physical activity are integral to the prevention and treatment of many types of health conditions is becoming accepted knowledge. The *SilverSneakers™ Fitness Program* is offered by leading Medicare health plans and Medicare Supplement carriers throughout the country (including Puerto Rico). More research indicates that physical inactivity is currently the biggest public health problem in this country and that the benefits of regular exercise and enhanced physical activity are not limited to heart, lungs and skeletal muscle, but may also include organs and tissues, such as the brain, liver, pancreas <u>and those in the inner ear</u>.[2]

Specific explanations of exercise frequency, intensity, type and time, also referred to as the FITT principle, have been provided as a result of hundreds if not thousands of studies, comparing a variety of exercise programs. Data from these comparative studies have resulted in the ACSM presenting the following evidence-based guidelines for exercise:

- Most adults should engage in moderate intensity cardiorespiratory exercise training for *equal to or greater than* [≥] 30 minutes per day on ≥5 days per week for a total of ≥150 minutes per week.
- Most adults should engage in vigorous intensity cardiorespiratory exercise training for ≥20 minutes per day on ≥3 days per week (≥75 minutes per week).
- Or they should engage in a combination of moderate and vigorous intensity exercise to achieve a total energy expenditure of ≥500-1000 MET•minutes per week (explained next).

METS (or metabolic equivalents) are units of energy expenditure. One MET is the energy expended at rest. Three METS is the energy expended during brisk walking at approximately 3 miles per hour (mph). If a person walks at 3 mph for 30 minutes, this is equivalent to 3 METS X 30 minutes = 90 MET•minutes. Six days per week of this type of physical activity would meet ACSM's recommended energy expenditure of ≥500-1000 MET•minutes per week.

On 2-3 days per week, adults should also perform resistance exercises for each of the major muscle groups, and neuromotor exercise involving balance, agility and coordination. Flexibility exercises for each of the major muscle-tendon groups (a total of 60 seconds per exercise) on ≥2 days per week are also recommended.[3] Of all the types of exercises that ACSM recommend, improvements in CV health and caloric energy expenditure that result in healthier body compositions (exercises that change the body shape) are the only proven mechanisms associated with exercise <u>that positively</u> <u>impact hearing sensitivity</u>. Improvements in muscle strength and flexibility, balance, agility and coordination have not been shown to benefit hearing.

Relationship between Exercise, CV Health and Hearing

Although CV health and fitness are known to have a genetic component, most research indicates that at least half of one's CV health and fitness is determined by lifestyle and environment, and is therefore controllable to a large extent. Exercising to music from external speakers or headsets gained popularity in the 1970s and 1980s as many people actively responded to the positive news about exercise and CV health. They participated in exercise classes and moved to the music of a variety of genres and loudness. Exercise workout tapes evolved into portable MP3 players, providing even more flexibility for exercising while listening to one's favorite tunes virtually anywhere. In the midst of these popular music workouts that gained a large following in the 1980s, audiologist Richard Navarro warned that listening to loud music while exercising might exacerbate the risk of hearing loss because of the exercise-induced redistribution of blood from the inner ear to the working muscles, leaving organs and tissues in the inner ear vulnerable to low oxygen levels.[4] His hypothesis initiated experiments, a few supporting the notion that any type of stress that increased heart rate dramatically (such as exercise), regardless of whether it included noise, contributed to temporary hearing loss. One of the first studies to investigate the association between hearing sensitivity and exercise found that when an acute bout of exercise was accompanied by noise exposure, a greater amount of temporary hearing loss occurred (compared against a resting state while in the presence of noise).[5] The conclusion that one exercise session accompanied by noise resulted in hearing loss <u>was not supported</u> by follow-up experiments.

The first published study that investigated regular exercise and hearing acuity was conducted by Ishmail and his researchers in 1973.[6] They reported improved hearing in subjects who participated in an unstructured exercise program for 20 weeks. Given these conflicting results, we challenged Navarro's theory as well as the few studies that appeared to support his work. When we conducted experiments that carefully controlled for exercise intensity, fitness level and specific noise exposure for a set time, our laboratory could not replicate his early results. In fact, we found that one bout of exercise alone did not alter hearing. Only when subjects were exposed to high-level noise, regardless whether they were sitting or exercising, were changes in hearing observed. Furthermore, like Ishmail's study, we found that persons who exercised regularly had better hearing than those who were sedentary.

Over the past 30 years, it has become clear that CV health and fitness positively impact hearing. Results from different laboratories across the country have shown that compared to low-fit individuals, persons with high CV health and fitness, particularly after age 50, maintain better hearing well into old age.[6-11] As researchers began to understand the role of sensory receptors in the nerve responsible for hearing, the relationship between the CV system and hearing ability became an increasingly popular topic. Exercise is positively correlated with improved blood circulation, prevention of neurotransmitter loss and less noise-induced hearing loss.[12] These changes in the vascular system allow improved blood circulation into different parts of the ear including the stria vascularis in the cochlea. This is important because the stria vascularis relies on adequate blood flow to function properly. Without constant replenishment of blood flow to the sensory receptors in the nerve of hearing, hearing ability could be compromised. Cardiovascular fitness may also help to preserve the way in which the central nervous system interprets speech (known as *central auditory processing*; see Chapter Three, Q&A#3). It has been found that CV fitness may reduce neurotransmitter loss associated with aging and thus preserve central auditory processing.[12]

Most certainly, the steady accumulation of scientific knowledge about the processes that protect hearing is the basis for developing successful treatments. We reported the positive effects of fitness on hearing with acute exercise and CV changes in 1994.[8] The study divided 28 healthy volunteers (average age 26) into three groups based on their fitness levels—high, moderate and low. All participants had normal hearing when the study began. The researchers exposed each group to three different noise levels that are similar to what one experiences in daily life (like traffic, power mowers, vacuum cleaners, noisy toys and amplified music). Hearing was re-evaluated under three different conditions:

- after 10 minutes of noise
- after vigorously riding a stationary bike for 10 minutes without noise
- and after listening to noise and exercising on the stationary bike at the same time.

During all three conditions, researchers also monitored heart rate, blood pressure and core body temperature. <u>The high-fit group consistently demonstrated better hearing levels in all cases</u> as compared to the low-fit group. Hearing levels for the moderately fit group fell right in the middle. Exposure to various noise levels produced more temporary hearing loss in the low-fit group than in the other two groups (see Chapter Three, Q&A#6). The findings suggest that moderate and high levels of CV fitness may protect against hearing loss. Low-fit individuals showed the poorest hearing acuity of all groups.

It's believed that regular exercise reduces susceptibility to temporary threshold shift referred to as TTS (poorer hearing) by increasing blood flow and oxygen delivery throughout the body, <u>including the ear</u>. Regardless of whether it's caused by micro- or macrovascular pathology, insufficient cochlear blood supply can disrupt the chemical balance of the inner ear fluid (endolymph) that in turn affects the electrical activity of the hair cells and, subsequently, activation of the auditory nerve.

<u>By improving circulation of oxygenated blood, the organ for hearing (cochlea) is less susceptible to the onset of vasoconstriction (narrowing of veins and arteries) brought on by loud noise</u>. Regular exercise keeps blood supply and oxygen flowing at optimal levels to cells and auditory nerve fibers in the ear. Noise, not acute exercise, was responsible for causing temporary hearing loss at virtually all frequencies between 2000 Hz and 8000 Hz.

While evidence from multiple studies got exercise off the hook for causing hearing loss, further inquiry resulted in an unexpected finding. Subjects with very healthy CV fitness levels (as evidenced by high VO_2max values for their age) also had the best hearing levels at nearly every frequency.[8] Remember that VO_2max is the maximum amount of oxygen that a person can breathe in with their lungs, pump out with their heart, and send via blood to their working muscles for energy requirements during a maximal physical effort. The ability to improve hearing with a CV fitness program that followed the FITT (frequency, intensity, type and time) principle was also investigated by us.[13] *Aerobic* simply means requiring air. The goal of aerobic exercise is to condition the heart and lungs to increase oxygen intake, transport and use by the body. In this study, subjects exercised at 70 percent of their aerobic capacity for 30 minutes, three days per week for two months. Ideally, we all should be getting this minimum exercise every week. It's important to understand that it's not required to break a sweat in order to undertake an aerobic exercise. An increase of 15-25 percent in VO_2max in these subjects (which moved them from a low-fit category to a moderate-fit category) correlated with improved hearing with the most improvement occurring at 2000 and 4000 Hz. This led to the conclusion that regular, moderate intensity exercise resulted in improved CV health and fitness and enhanced hearing as well. Additional benefits derived were improved reflex reactions and better ability to read newsprint without eyeglasses for some subjects. These results demonstrate the plasticity of hearing acuity as well as the CV system; that is, the ability of both systems to change for the better as a result of a positive lifestyle intervention, regardless of age.

What may also be important is the production of heat shock proteins. These are substances scientists believe help minimize damage throughout the body. Research in cellular mechanisms in the cochlea revealed that cells under stress from noise, ototoxic drugs and aging, generate these proteins to protect surviving cells. Several laboratories have demonstrated positive protective pharmacological effects of specific proteins against cochlear damage.[14] The inner ear (cochlea) contains 17,500 to 23,500 hair follicles referred to as sensory *hair cells.* They're called hair cells because that's what they look like (see Chapter Three, Q&A#5, image Figures 3-1 and 3-2). The observations that hair cells contain specific proteins that undergo changes in structure with slight swelling suggest that active elements exist to protect tissue from damage. Such proteins may also play key roles in protecting hair cells from metabolic and aging changes. Also, antioxidant research has allowed scientists to better understand the effects of certain nutrients on circulation within the ear. Results of one study using folic acid (which scavenges free radical molecules) demonstrated that participants who supplemented their diet with this protein for 3 years evidenced improvement in low-frequency hearing.[15] There is evidence that people who are more fit have more of these heat shock proteins that in turn could explain how regular exercise may help protect hearing from everyday noise damage.

In another study, improved hearing was observed in older adults with high cardiovascular health and fitness; however, a surprising finding defined specific types of fitness associated with gains and losses in hearing acuity. Adults who had high muscle strength but low CV health had poorer hearing.[16] Based on these results of a cross-sampling of individuals, we recommend that CV exercise be included either alone or in conjunction with strength training as a contributor to preserve and possibly enhance hearing in adults of varying ages. Persons in their 20s, 30s and 40s maintained good general hearing ability, regardless of fitness level (Figure 6-2). However after age 50, persons with medium and high CV fitness consistently showed better hearing at high frequencies than persons of the same age with low CV fitness.

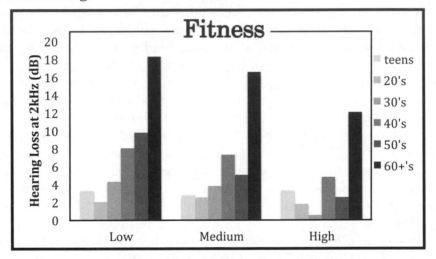

Figure 6-2: the higher the cardiovascular fitness (shown as low, medium and high), the better the hearing acuity in most age groups

After the association between hearing, age and CV fitness was established, we then conducted a longitudinal study of 25 people between the ages of 12 and 76 tested twice over a five-year period.[17] Our goal was to determine if CV fitness and hearing acuity changed in a similar way over time. That is, we wanted to observe if young low-fit individuals demonstrated poorer hearing five years later, and if young, moderate- or high-fit individuals demonstrated better hearing five years later. Unlike a cross-sectional study, a longitudinal study follows the same subjects for a period of time and controls factors related to historical events or actions that may affect one group of people in a particular age group, but not another. Examples include different noise exposure levels in work settings.

Study participants were sorted into three CV fitness groups: high, medium and low; and conducted two test periods five years apart. During this testing, hearing acuity was compared using two measures: hearing thresholds (the softest level at which sound can be heard 50 percent of the time) and otoacoustic emissions (an internal feedback produced by ears when exposed to sound). Otoacoustic emission tests—the same ones used with newborn babies—specifically evaluate the sensory cells in the auditory nerve and can detect nerve damage before a significant hearing loss is present. Our results showed that unlike low-fit people whose hearing got worse five years later, people with high CV fitness maintained their hearing from the prior five years. This indicated that at the second testing, sound did not have to be any louder in order for them to hear it than it did when they were first tested. <u>This is a notable and desirable maintenance of hearing sensitivity over time</u>. Furthermore, individuals with high CV fitness during the first test session who maintained their CV fitness over the five years between testing had better hearing acuity over time than those who did not maintain CV fitness or who had low CV.

An important conclusion from virtually all of these experiments is not just that high cardiovascular fitness is correlated with better hearing sensitivity, but also that adults with the lowest level of CV fitness virtually always had poorer hearing. This was also evident when considering an individual's age and gender, indicating that <u>CV fitness has a protective effect on hearing as a person ages</u>. The relationship between CV fitness and hearing was confirmed in a national study on hearing sensitivity using data collected from the 1999-2004 National Health and Nutrition Examination Survey. The study included 1,082 participants representative of 42,869,850 adults between the ages of 20 and 49. It found that compared to low-fit individuals, males as well as females with good hearing had higher VO_2max values.[12] The correlation between exercise and hearing was particularly strong for female participants. These females with high cardiovascular fitness levels were also found to have better hearing at lower frequencies as well as higher frequencies. These findings indicate that cardiovascular health is a powerful influence over hearing sensitivity, and individuals with high CV fitness can maintain better hearing acuity well into adulthood, while persons with low CV fitness are likely to have poorer hearing.

Body Composition and Hearing

In addition to biomarkers for cardiovascular health and fitness, VO$_2$max, and blood pressure (another component of fitness), body composition has been shown to be associated with hearing acuity.[9] Body composition can be assessed in many different ways, including weight alone, height to weight ratio, percent fat, percent lean body mass, waist circumference, and waist-to-hip circumference ratios. The goal of these measurements is to determine if a person is a healthy weight for their height, underweight, overweight, or obese. Being underweight is a risk factor for frailty and degenerative diseases, such as osteoporosis and cancer. The majority of Americans are overweight or at risk for being obese due to lifestyles of physical inactivity and overconsumption of food. Conditions of being overweight or obese are directly associated with many age-related diseases including heart disease, diabetes, arthritis, and certain types of cancer. Typically, people who are overweight are also less physically active than those with healthy body weight, which may explain the usual lower cardiovascular health and fitness of overweight individuals. Being overweight typically refers to excessive body weight relative to height. While some people use subjective ways (e.g., How do my clothes fit? How do I feel?) to estimate whether they are too fat or too thin, the more popular and accurate way to assess body composition is by using height and weight data to calculate body mass index (BMI). For readers interested in this formula, BMI is represented by weight in pounds divided by height in inches, squared (height X height) and multiplied by 703. For example, if you weigh 140 pounds and are 5 foot 5 inches tall, your BMI would be calculated as 140 ÷ (65 X 65) X 703 = BMI. 140 ÷ 4225 x 703 = 23.3. Another option is to use a chart that incorporates this formula into a wide selection of heights and weights (see Figure 6-3) to provide BMI values.

Healthy BMI values range from approximately 19-25 and depend on the proportion of weight for one's height to get a sense for being under or overweight depending on height. However, BMI values are not the same as percent body fat. Obesity specifically refers to excessive body fat, often measured by bioelectrical impedance, skin fold calipers or air displacement (among others). Women with total body fat over 30 percent and men with total body fat over 25 percent are considered to be obese. It should come as no surprise that compared to adults who have healthy body compositions, adults who are either overweight or obese suffer from more diseases, including hypertension, hyperlipidemia, and diabetes. In the past decade, evidence has emerged that waist circumference is a powerful predictor of obesity risk and that when coupled with BMI, both waist circumference and BMI predict health risk, including premature death, better than BMI alone.[18] This intriguing finding (that a measurement as simple and low cost as waist and/or hip circumference can be such a powerful indicator for health and disease) is finding its way into physicians' offices across the country, as part of routine health screening.

Preliminary data from our laboratory indicates that body composition is an important health-related component associated with hearing sensitivity. Specifically, BMI is inversely related to hearing sensitivity. That is, the higher the BMI, the poorer the hearing acuity. In a study of 67 middle-age adults, individuals who were classified with normal BMI levels had normal hearing, while those with BMI values classified as obese had poorer hearing at 8000 Hz.[19] Figure 6-3 (page 126) shows a color chart for determining BMI based on height and weight with designated risk zones.

BMI is not a direct measure of body fat, nor does it provide a map for where fat is distributed around the body. Nevertheless, body mass index has been shown in some studies to correlate directly with risk for the cardiovascular rate of disease (morbidity) and mortality.[20] That is, the higher the number, the greater the risk of CV disease. In a recent study of college-age students, a trend was observed whereby the higher the body mass index, the worse the hearing acuity.

Waist-to-hip measurements provide more information regarding fat topography and provide a better geographic map on where body fat is distributed. "Apples" (the people who store more fat centrally or in the abdominal area) have been reported to be at higher risk for developing heart disease and type 2 diabetes.[21-22] Of particular interest in our preliminary studies, waist-to-hip ratio is observed to be inversely related to hearing in a similar way as body mass index. That is, individuals having more of an "apple" body shape had poorer hearing when compared with "pear" body shapes or healthier BMI and waist-to-hip values. This simple no-cost method of assessing health using waist and/or hip circumference measurements may be a valuable biomarker for obesity, cardiovascular disease, metabolic disease, as well as hearing loss. Take advantage of Figure 6-4 (on page 127) to determine your risk.

Figure 6-3: Body Mass Index Chart

Body Mass Index Chart

Weight in Pounds (100 to 250)

Height in Inches	100	110	120	130	140	150	160	170	180	190	200	210	220	230	240	250
48	30.5	33.6	36.6	39.7	42.7	45.8	48.8	51.9	54.9	58.0	61.0	64.1	67.1	70.2	73.2	76.3
50	28.1	30.9	33.7	36.6	39.4	42.2	45.0	47.8	50.6	53.4	56.2	59.1	61.9	64.7	67.5	70.3
52	26.0	28.6	31.2	33.8	36.4	39.0	41.6	44.2	46.8	49.4	52.0	54.6	57.2	59.8	62.4	65.0
54	24.1	26.5	28.9	31.3	33.8	36.2	38.6	41.0	43.4	45.8	48.2	50.6	53.0	55.4	57.9	60.3
56	22.4	24.7	26.9	29.1	31.4	33.6	35.9	38.1	40.4	42.6	44.8	47.1	49.3	51.6	53.8	56.0
58	20.9	23.0	25.1	27.2	29.3	31.3	33.4	35.5	37.6	39.7	41.8	43.9	46.0	48.1	50.2	52.2
60	19.5	21.5	23.4	25.4	27.3	29.3	31.2	33.2	35.2	37.1	39.1	41.0	43.0	44.9	46.9	48.8
62	18.3	20.1	21.9	23.8	25.6	27.4	29.3	31.1	32.9	34.7	36.6	38.4	40.2	42.1	43.9	45.7
64	17.2	18.9	20.6	22.3	24.0	25.7	27.5	29.2	30.9	32.6	34.3	36.0	37.8	39.5	41.2	42.9
66	16.1	17.8	19.4	21.0	22.6	24.2	25.8	27.4	29.0	30.7	32.3	33.9	35.5	37.1	38.7	40.3
68	15.2	16.7	18.2	19.8	21.3	22.8	24.3	25.8	27.4	28.9	30.4	31.9	33.4	35.0	36.5	38.0
70	14.3	15.8	17.2	18.7	20.1	21.5	23.0	24.4	25.8	27.3	28.7	30.1	31.6	33.0	34.4	35.9
72	13.6	14.9	16.3	17.6	19.0	20.3	21.7	23.1	24.4	25.8	27.1	28.5	29.8	31.2	32.5	33.9
74	12.8	14.1	15.4	16.7	18.0	19.3	20.5	21.8	23.1	24.4	25.7	27.0	28.2	29.5	30.8	32.1
76	12.2	13.4	14.6	15.8	17.0	18.3	19.5	20.7	21.9	23.1	24.3	25.6	26.8	28.0	29.2	30.4
78	11.6	12.7	13.9	15.0	16.2	17.3	18.5	19.6	20.8	22.0	23.1	24.3	25.4	26.6	27.7	28.9
80	11.0	12.1	13.2	14.3	15.4	16.5	17.6	18.7	19.8	20.9	22.0	23.1	24.2	25.3	26.4	27.5
82	10.5	11.5	12.5	13.6	14.6	15.7	16.7	17.8	18.8	19.9	20.9	22.0	23.0	24.0	25.1	26.1
84	10.0	11.0	12.0	13.0	13.9	14.9	15.9	16.9	17.9	18.9	19.9	20.9	21.9	22.9	23.9	24.9

< 18.5 Underweight | 18.5-24.9 Normal | 25.0-29.9 Overweight | 30.0 or > Obesity

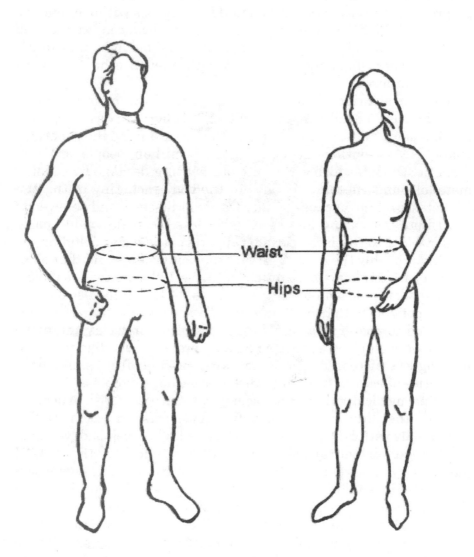

Figure 6-4: waist and hip circumference in women and men

Factors Contributing to Hearing Loss other than Noise

A number of health and inheritance factors contribute to the progression and severity of individual hearing loss within or outside our control. They range from genetics and medical conditions, such as diabetes, cancer and HIV, to personality and behavioral factors.[23] In some cases, hearing loss occurs with age; in other cases it's observed at birth.

The prevalence of diabetes mellitus in the U.S. in both children and adults is 25.8 million people, with 1.9 million new cases reported in 2010 alone. Most disconcerting is that according to the American Diabetes Association, an additional 79 million people are pre-diabetic. Diabetes also contributes to hearing damage by causing metabolic and vascular changes in the body including in the ear. Diabetes is a known cause of microvascular disease, and believed to contribute to hearing loss by causing less blood flow and poorer quality blood to reach the peripheral parts of the body, including the ear and probably the eyes. A recent study on vision found that older women with damage to the retina (retinopathy) were twice as likely to have hearing loss in lower frequencies.[24] This study also showed that in patients with hearing loss and diabetes, *worsening creatinine levels* led to poorer hearing. That is, as blood, muscles and urine became less efficient at dumping waste products, the likelihood for hearing loss increased. Therefore, cardiovascular fitness may have protective effects on the rate of diseases such as diabetes.

A final medical condition associated with increased risk of hearing loss is the human immunodeficiency virus infection (HIV). Individuals with HIV are shown to have a higher risk of developing sudden sensorineural hearing loss than those without HIV, particularly males between the ages of 18 to 35. And this population is more than two times more likely to develop sensorineural hearing loss than those in the general population without HIV.[25]

Personality is another non-acoustic factor that may contribute to hearing loss. In general, it has been found that <u>individuals who are more prone to stress may be more likely to develop temporary hearing loss</u> than those who are less stress-prone when presented with the same amount of noise exposure. This was confirmed in a research study in which individuals were sorted into two groups: the Type A (coronary-prone) group consisted of individuals who tended to have higher reactions to stress, and the Type B (non-coronary prone) group. Studies have found that <u>Type A personalities tend to have longer periods of peripheral blood vessel constriction</u> leading to reduced blood circulation in the inner ear. In other words, when you tense your body, you tend to reduce blood flow. This might mean sensing a bit of numbness in your extremities, colder fingers, muscle ache or cramps, or a sense of fatigue. This reduced circulation placed the individuals at a higher risk for developing temporary hearing loss than their Type B personality counterparts.

A similar study confirmed the relationship between hearing loss and stress. They found that Type A (coronary-prone) personalities had poorer hearing levels at specific tones following 10 minutes of noise, and following 10 minutes of noise accompanied by exercise than did their Type B counterparts.[23] The changes in temporary hearing sensitivity in the Type A personality group occurred independent of differences in circulatory and heart rate measures (compared with the control group) following either noise, or noise and exercise. These studies indicate that stress factors other than increased heart rate and blood pressure contribute to TTS. Permanent threshold shift represents the most common hearing effect of medical factors and loud noise, and is related to a number of factors including the number of exposures and exposure duration. From this discussion, it's apparent that several different medical and personality factors may contribute to hearing loss.

What You Can Do

As you continue to age, knowledge of many factors that influence hearing sensitivity, especially those that can be modified, may empower you to adjust certain aspects of your lifestyle to generate a positive influence on life quality and life expectancy. In addition to adding aerobic exercise to your life as explained in this chapter, you can also purchase a pedometer to track your number of footsteps (or mileage) to be sure you're attaining the desirable targets. If you want to exercise or walk to the sound of music, keep the volume at a level where you can hear someone within arm's reach speaking to you. Pay close attention to your body weight and fat storage by monitoring your BMI and waist and hip circumference. Obesity and "apple" shapes where excess fat is stored in the abdominal region add to risk for CV disease and hearing loss. Find ways to reduce stress in your life and increase your ability to stay calm regardless of your personality type. In the words of Kofi Annan, information can be liberating, since it can spring you into action with the assistance of healthcare professionals, to undergo appropriate interventions designed to maintain or improve your life, and subsequently provide you with more healthy, productive and even happier years.

References

1. Moyer VA. (2012). Screening for hearing loss in older adults: U.S. preventive service task force recommendation statement. *Annals in Internal Medicine,* 157: 655-661.

2. Blair SN. (2009). Physical inactivity: The biggest public health problem of the 21st century. *British Journal of Sports Medicine,* 43: 1-2.

3. Garber CE, Blissmer B, Deschennes MR, et al. (2011). American college of sports medicine position stand. Quantity and quality of exercise for developing and maintaining cardiorespiratory, musculoskeletal, and neuromotor fitness in apparently healthy adults: Guidance for prescribing exercise. *Medicine and Science in Sports and Exercise,* 43:1334-59.

4. Navarro R. (1990). Sports scan. *Physician and Sports Medicine,* 18, 6.

5. Saxon SA & Dahle AJ. (1971). Auditory threshold variations during periods of induced high and low heart rates. *Psycho-physiology,* 8: 23-29.

6. Ishmail AH, Corrigan DL, MacLeod DF, et al. (1973). Biophysiological and audiological variables in adults. *Archives in Otolaryngology,* 97: 447-451.

7. Alessio HM & Hutchinson KM. (1991). Effects of submaximal exercise and noise exposure on hearing loss. *Research Quarterly for Exercise and Sports,* 62: 413-9.

8. Manson J, Alessio HM, Cristell M. (1994). Does cardiovascular health mediate hearing ability? *Medicine and Science in Sports and Exercise,* 26: 866-871.

9. Kolkhorst FW, Smaldino JJ, Wolf SC, et al. (1998). Influence of fitness on susceptibility to noise-induced temporary threshold shift. *Medicine and Science in Sports and Exercise,* 30: 289-93.

10. Agrawal Y, Platz EA & Niparko JK. (2008). Prevalence of hearing loss and differences by demographic characteristics among US adults: Data from the National Health and Nutrition Examination Survey, 1999-2004. *Archives of Internal Medicine,* 168: 1522-1530.

11. Hutchinson KM, Alessio HM & Baiduc RR. (2010). Association between cardiovascular health and hearing function: Pure-tone and

distortion product otoacoustic emission measures. *American Journal of Audiology,* 19: 26-35.

12. Hull RH & Kerschen SR. (2010). The influence of cardiovascular health on peripheral and central auditory function in adults: a research review. *American Journal of Audiology,* 19: 9-16.

13. Cristell M, Hutchinson KM & Alessio, HM. (1998). Effects of exercise training on hearing ability. *Scandinavian Audiology,* 27, 219-224.

14. Taleb M, Braondon CS., Lee F-S, et al. (2009). Hsp70 inhibits aminoglycoside-induced hearing loss and cochlear hair cell death. *Cell Stress Chaparones,* 14: 427-437.

15. Durga J, Verhoef P, Anteunis L J, et al. (2007). Effects of folic acid supplementation on hearing in older adults: a randomized, controlled trial. *Annals of Internal Medicine,* 146: 1–9.

16. Hutchinson KM, Alessio HM, Hoppes S, et al. (2000). Effects of cardiovascular fitness and muscle strength on hearing sensitivity. *Journal of Strength and Conditioning Research,* 14: 302-309.

17. Alessio HM & Hutchinson KM. (2004). Exercise promotes hearing health. *The Hearing Review,* Retrieved from http://www.hearingreview.com/all-news/15862-exercise-promotes-hearing-health.

18. Janssen I, Katzmarzyk PT, & Ross R. (2004). Waist circumference and not body mass index explains obesity-related health risk. *American Journal of Clinical Nutrition,* 79: 379-384.

19. Wagner S, Lenzini S, Wharton T, et al. (2013, March). "Personal listening device use, hearing, health and fitness." Poster session presented at the annual convention of the Ohio Speech Language and Hearing Association, Columbus, OH.

20. Frankel S, Elwood P, Smith GD, et al. (1996). Birthweight, body mass index in middle age, and incident coronary heart disease. *The Lancet,* 348: 1478-1580.

21. Jacobs EJ, Newton CC, Wang Y, et al. (2010). Waist circumference and all-cause mortality in a large US cohort. *Archives of Internal Medicine,* 170: 1293-1301.

22. Despres JP, Lemieux I, & Prud'homme D. (2001).Treatment of obesity: Need to focus on high risk abdominally obese patients. *British Medical Journal,* 322: 716-720.

23. Hutchinson K, & Alessio HM. (1996). Influence of personality type on susceptibility to the effects of noise exposure. *Journal of Psychological Type,* 39: 30-36.

24. Kakarlapudi V, Sawyer R & Staecker H. (2003). The effect of diabetes on sensorineural hearing loss. *Otology and Neurotology,* 24: 382–386.

25. Lin C, Lin S, Weng S, et al. (2013). Increased risk of sudden sensorineural hearing loss in patients with human immuno-deficiency virus aged 18 to 35 years: A population-based cohort study. *Journal of the American Medical Association Otolaryngology Head Neck Surgery,* 139: 251-255.

CHAPTER SEVEN
Why Some Consumers Reject Hearing Aids But How You Could Love Them!

Sergei Kochkin, PhD

Recent research in the United States indicates that close to 35 million people have a hearing loss they are aware of—approximately 11 percent of Americans.[1] If we include 13 million people with tinnitus, who are not aware of their underlying hearing loss, then the figure is probably closer to 48 million Americans with hearing loss.[2] In addition, about 1.1 million school-age children have a hearing loss. The early identification and treatment of hearing loss in children are particularly critical because normal development of speech and language depend on hearing. It's important that you understand the prevalence of hearing loss and the fact that it cuts across all age groups. In fact, most people are amazed when they learn that 60 percent of people with hearing loss are below retirement age.[1] In focus groups with people who have rejected hearing aids, some people with hearing loss expressed the erroneous conclusions that they are rare or obscure individuals, "since so few people have hearing loss" or that their hearing loss "is a sign of aging." When shown that they were not alone and that most people with hearing loss are younger than they were, they tended to be more accepting of their hearing loss and therefore more willing to seek a hearing aid solution.

Conversations with experts in other countries generally recognize that close to 10 percent of the populations in developed countries have problems with their hearing. I happen to believe the actual figure may be higher, because most studies have not included hearing loss populations in institutional settings such as nursing or retirement homes, the military, and prisons.

The vast majority can be helped by hearing aids. Because of major breakthroughs in hearing aid technology in recent years, we can now do a better job of matching technology with a candidate's lifestyle and communication needs. Yet, some purchased hearing aids still end up in their owners' drawers, unworn.[3] The good news is that many of the problems with hearing aids have been solved, and wearers can now expect improved communication with hearing aids as the rule, not the exception.

Why do some individuals have difficulty adjusting to hearing aids while others are doing so well that people around them don't even notice they're wearing them? What's different about successful hearing aid wearers? And why do only one in five individuals with hearing loss use hearing aids despite the proven value of amplification? Some interesting facts now coming to light may answer these questions.

Why Some People Reject Hearing Aids

More than 24 million people in the United States with hearing loss have chosen not to adopt hearing aids as a solution. Two research investigations polled close to 6,000 individuals with self-reported hearing loss regarding their reluctance to try hearing aids or factors that may expedite adoption of hearing aids.[4-5] Here are some of the reasons why consumers have declined to pursue them.

1. Inadequate Information

Many people are not aware they have a hearing loss and therefore are in need of information that would help them recognize it. Most people lose hearing gradually. In most cases, it's slowly progressive. During this time, both the person with hearing loss and family members adapt to it, often not even realizing that they're doing this. The number one reason why people buy their very first hearing aid is the "recognition that their hearing got worse;" usually this means they made embarrassing mistakes in social settings due to their untreated hearing loss. Thus, one of the first things individuals with suspected hearing loss should do is determine if they exhibit some of the signs of hearing loss. The Better Hearing Institute has validated a reliable online hearing check on 11,000 subjects that would enable you to determine the probable extent of your hearing loss (see www.hearingcheck.org).

2. Stigma and Cosmetics

Some people reject hearing aids because they're concerned with the stigma of hearing loss or are in a state of denial, and thus they try to hide it from others. It's unfortunate, but many people, because they have less than perfect hearing, believe they are inferior, unintelligent, or simply less lovable. They believe other people will think they're getting older or will view them as less competent, less attractive, and so on. They may have shame regarding their hearing loss. This is partly due to the fact that we live in a youth-oriented, airbrushed society that stresses physical perfection as an important human attribute.

As you previously read in this book, cosmetics no longer need to be a barrier to obtaining amplification. Since the 1990s, technological advances have permitted the hearing aid industry to develop hearing instruments like CIC hearing aids or the new open fit, which are virtually invisible (see Chapter 4, Figure 4-1). In fact, research shows that 90 percent of consumers perceived these hearing aids to be completely invisible. Based on your hearing needs and the physical characteristics of your ears, you might be a candidate for these "invisible" devices. If you're not, rest assured that in-the-canal (ITC) devices, although larger, are available to fit many hearing losses and are discreetly hidden.

Understand though, that once you begin hearing through amplification and once it has enhanced your quality of life, cosmetics will be of lesser concern to you. Research shows that people who have come to enjoy their hearing aids rate even the largest hearing aids as cosmetically appealing as compared to some of the smaller, in-the-ear models.[6] Some hearing instruments even come in bright colors—dispelling the myth that they're something to be ashamed of or hide! So, stigma and cosmetic concerns of the past five years are now substantially diminished, and for most who wear them, completely resolved.

3. Misdirected Medical Guidance

Many people have received misinformation from well-intending physicians about their hearing loss and the extent to which it can be helped. For instance, many physicians have advised their patients that they're not candidates for hearing aids if they have hearing loss in one ear and good hearing in the other (unilateral hearing loss); if they have "nerve deafness" (an obsolete term for sensorineural hearing loss); or if the hearing loss still allows them to conduct a conversation in quiet. Many times, the doctor's opinion will derive from the fact that the patient and doctor are able to conduct a face-to-face conversation in the secluded and usually quiet exam room. Much of this unintentional misinformation comes from family physicians who don't specialize in hearing problems. In fact, most physicians (except ENT specialists) receive very little training in medical school in the areas of hearing loss and hearing aids. The only helpful information will come from those who specialize in hearing loss.

Another reason for rejection of hearing aids is that people have forgotten how important hearing is to their quality of life. We live in such a visually oriented society that often hearing plays a secondary role. As you know from your own experience or from this book, people who cannot hear well often have lives filled with anxiety, insecurity, isolation, and depression. People gradually withdraw from family and friends because without auditory contact they lose the feeling of being connected. In essence, they grow numb to the world around them. But in the real world (or as Dr. Carmen suggested, "the outside world,") interpersonal communication is critical.

A significant number of people with hearing loss mistakenly believe that hearing aids are not effective for what they're designed to do. Many people judge hearing aids based on what they've seen their grandparents wear—a large, clunky box about the size of a pack of cigarettes with wires coming out of it.

Recent research with consumers utilizing a variety of hearing aids (high technology as well as older technology aids 1-5 years old) indicated that 86 percent of hearing aid wearers reported satisfaction (defined as *somewhat satisfied, satisfied,* or *very satisfied*) with the ability of the hearing aids to improve their hearing, and 75 percent reported that hearing aids have improved the quality of their life. A significant number of people reported satisfaction with their hearing aids in quiet situations (91 percent) as well as in very difficult situations such as restaurants (75 percent), places of worship (75 percent), or large groups (68 percent).

In research with more than 35,000 consumers, I've learned that not everyone benefits equally in all listening situations, nor do all types of hearing aid circuitry perform the same in difficult listening situations. For example, the average hearing aid achieves a 61 percent satisfaction rating in noisy situations; yet some technologies, notably programmable hearing aids with multiple microphones (known as *directional* hearing aids), have achieved significantly higher satisfaction ratings. With the advent of wireless technology, giving the consumer connectivity to cell phones, televisions and stereos, and even companion wireless microphones, we would expect consumer satisfaction to increase more as the sound source is piped directly into the consumer's hearing aid.

Also, only about 69 percent of consumers are satisfied with hearing aids on the telephone, yet some instruments, such as CIC hearing aids, perform better on the phone as well as outdoors because they're located just inside the entrance of the ear canal and produce less feedback while on the phone. Much of this satisfaction may also be due to diminished wind noises outdoors, a sense of more natural amplification, and the need for somewhat less power, resulting in increased tolerance of background noise.[6-9] Understand that hearing aids in the "Telephone" mode completely eliminate feedback (see Chapter 6 and Appendix I).

In the last several years, smaller behind-the-ear open fit hearing aids have become the rage in America. They have solved some of the long-term complaints of consumers: the sound of their voice is more natural, and it no longer feels as if they're hearing in a barrel (occlusion); the fit is more comfortable because their hearing aid shell is not in their ear; it is in fact less visible than in-the-ear (ITE) devices; there's less whistling and feedback; the sound quality is more natural; and wearers believe they're achieving more benefit.[8]

Since the digital revolution, now close to 100 percent of hearing aids sold in America are digital. Have digital hearing aids improved the consumer's experience? Our recent survey with close to 2,000 consumers of hearing aids associated the use of digital hearing instruments with significantly higher overall satisfaction and benefit; improved sound quality; reduction in feedback; improved performance in noisy situations; and greater utility in a number of important listening situations.[6] With continued advances in digital signal processing and the wireless revolution, I'm confident that the utility of hearing aids will improve dramatically in the next decade.

6. Failure to Trust in a Hearing Aid Dispensing Professional

Another reason some people hold off their purchase is: "I do not trust hearing health providers who fit hearing aids!" Yet, the data show that 93 percent of consumers felt satisfied with their hearing aid dispensing professional.[10] It's certainly worth mentioning that the training, education, and experience of dispensers of hearing aids have greatly increased over the years, for both audiologists and hearing instrument specialists (see Chapter 11).

7. Unrecognized Value of Hearing Aids

Many people who have avoided amplification tend to believe there's little value in hearing aids. They mistakenly assume that "hearing aids will not work for them" and therefore they will not derive any benefit. Both consumers and physicians have little knowledge of the potential benefit of hearing aids. Since the new millennium, large-scale research has examined the impact of hearing aids on quality of life for people who use hearing aids in the United States.[7,11]

In my humble opinion, I cannot think of a consumer product with such an impressive list of potential benefits: greater earning power; improved interpersonal relationships; reduced discrimination toward the person with the hearing loss; reduced difficulty in communicating; less need to compensate for hearing loss; reduced anger and frustration; reduction in depression and anxiety; enhanced emotional stability; reductions in paranoid feelings; reduced social phobias; greater belief that you are in control of your life; reduced self-criticism; increased self-esteem; improved perceptions of mental acuity; improved health status; greater level of outgoingness (e.g., extraversion); and greater likelihood of participating in groups. I challenge anyone to name a product or a service with this impressive list of benefits. When I presented these findings to a group of medical doctors, one prominent physician stated, "I was not aware of the seriousness of hearing loss and the potential for hearing aids to alleviate the problem. Every doctor in the world must be made aware of these findings!"

8. Feeling Priced Out of the Market

Some people with hearing loss simply do not have the disposable income that would enable them to afford today's modern hearing aids and healthcare treatment. Based on the known benefits of hearing aids improving quality of life, there's some effort being generated to see if more government programs such as Medicare will cover hearing aids. If the person with a hearing loss is a child, many local and state governments offer hearing aids at no or reduced cost. Check to see if you qualify for free aids or for a reduced price for hearing aids through your union, employer, the Veterans Administration, your insurance provider, your HMO, your local Lions Club. If you're still working see if you can qualify for pre-tax savings through your employer's medical flex-dollar health program. There's also a current initiative to provide a $500 tax credit per hearing aid for children, boomers, and seniors. To make your voice heard on this bill, visit www.hearingaidtaxcredit.org. Also listed are charitable foundations that provide help with hearing aids under "Resources" (Financial) at www.betterhearing.org.

Twelve Ways to Optimize Your Chances of being a Satisfied Hearing Aid Wearer

There is nothing more important to the manufacturers of hearing aids and hearing healthcare professionals than your satisfaction with their product and services. Like other smart professionals, they know that satisfied clients lead to repeat business and to positive word-of-mouth advertising for their products. The hearing aid industry is interested in delighting you, in meeting your needs and exceeding your expectations. The people-oriented hearing aid industry fosters significant interaction and communication between the person with hearing loss and hearing health professionals to assure that they've done all things possible to meet your needs. You have a role to play in assuring your satisfaction with hearing aids. So, I would like to offer some suggestions for optimizing the chances that you'll be one of these delighted hearing aid wearers.

1. Meeting Your Needs

Simply stated, satisfaction is having your needs, desires or expectations met. Another way of looking at satisfaction is feeling fulfilled; based on promises met by your hearing healthcare provider. You have very specific needs, and the purpose of the hearing healthcare provider is to find out what your needs are and how to meet them. Thus, during the process of rediscovering your hearing, it's important to determine what these needs are, what outcomes you're looking for, and most importantly, how you'll know when you've met your needs. The clearer you are about this, the more likely a positive outcome. Many people go to their hearing healthcare practitioner with a vague concept of their needs: "I can't hear," or "It seems as if people are mumbling more," or worse yet, "My wife says I don't listen to her."

I believe you will have a more fulfilling hearing aid experience if you dig deeper to comprehend the impact your hearing loss has had on you emotionally, behaviorally, mentally, and socially. A number of chapters in this book can help you meet this challenge. Write the issues down because they'll become a roadmap for both you and your hearing healthcare professional. Also, many hearing healthcare professionals have assessment scales that will help you understand problems caused by your hearing loss. Once you know your problems, you can better identify your expected outcomes. It's your personal needs list, and when it's fulfilled, it will bring a smile to your face and the faces of your loved ones. This list also becomes a contract between you and your hearing care professional.

2. Motivation

Advanced hearing aid technology can now compensate for most hearing losses, but millions of hearing aid candidates still are not ready to accept this fact. Is there a missing link? I think so. People with hearing loss are in different stages of readiness. At one extreme, the individual is in denial about the hearing loss. If either a family member or a professional insists on hearing aids at this point, behavior is unlikely to change, and most likely such a person would be dissatisfied if wearing hearing aids.

Individuals highly motivated to improve their hearing have an infinitely better chance of success with hearing aids. Such motivated people recognize their hearing loss and are open to change. They tend to seek relevant information related to their hearing loss and the technology needed to alleviate the hearing problem. The most highly motivated hearing aid candidates have a willingness to discuss their feelings about their hearing problem and explore some hearing options that might be available to them. When fit with hearing aids, they eagerly explore their new technology, discuss problems during follow-up visits with their hearing health professional, and patiently learn to adapt to their technology.

3. Positive Attitude

The most important personality trait that one could possess is a positive attitude, not just toward the process of obtaining hearing aids, but toward life in general. This means a willingness to try hearing aids, adapt to new solutions, and keep frustration at a minimum when obstacles arise. If you view your circumstances as beyond your control, there's a higher probability that you'll be less successful in adapting to change, including hearing aid use.

Hearing aid studies have shown that people who have a positive outlook on life do better with hearing aids.[12] They have a positive self-image and believe they're in control of their life. My recommendation is take charge and be determined to improve the quality of your life with today's modern hearing aids.

4. Age of Your Hearing Aids

It's human nature to want to keep your hearing aids as long as possible in order to maximize value. However, hearing aids do wear out over time, ear canals change in shape, and the pattern of your hearing loss is likely to change in time. In the research that I've conducted, customer satisfaction was at its highest in the first year of use (78 percent). After five years of use, satisfaction dropped significantly to 58 percent, and after ten years of use even lower to 51 percent.[13]

So, it's important that you make sure that both the physical and audiological fit of your hearing aids is optimized for your hearing loss today rather than the way it was five, ten, or fifteen years ago. I would recommend that you replace your hearing aids every five years (if affordable) or when there have been significant advances in technology.

5. Choice of Technology

I've conducted extensive research across dozens of technologies. There is no doubt that customers are more satisfied with programmable, digital, and directional technology. Advanced digital technology allows the dispenser to adjust the hearing aid to your specific hearing loss characteristics with more precision. If the product does not meet your needs, then the hearing healthcare professional can adjust the hearing aid at the office versus sending it back to the manufacturer for adjustment.

With advancements in hearing aid technology has come a corresponding improvement in computer software that acoustically fits your hearing instruments to your specific needs. For example, some manufacturers store hundreds of real world sounds in the computer and allow you to see how your hearing aids will sound in those situations. This tremendous feature allows the hearing care practitioner to dynamically adjust the hearing aids based on your personal reaction to sounds.

A second advanced feature to consider is directional hearing aids. They have two microphones in them. Because of their design, they're able to reduce some annoying background noise and improve your ability to understand speech in many difficult listening situations. Conducting three studies on directional hearing aids, I found a 17 percent customer satisfaction improvement in two studies and a 26 percent improvement in another.[9,14] The latter achieved a 90 percent customer satisfaction rating, the highest I have ever seen for a hearing aid. If you're an active person, then directional hearing aids could be suitable for you.

Finally, consider purchasing wireless or Bluetooth compatible hearing aids if you can afford them. Wireless accessories can help you in more challenging listening situations and provide added performance capability giving you greater access to listening situations that are important to you. Many hearing aid manufacturers offer a companion wireless microphone that can be used in several ways. It can be given to a significant other in the car or at a restaurant, for example. The significant other wears it on their shirt or blouse and their voice is picked up by the microphone and sent straight to the hearing aid or with a neck-worn relay device. This improves the signal-to-noise ratio for the wearer and helps to compensate for distance and noise. These marvels of technology also allow you to connect to your MP3 player, your stereo or TV and your cell phone. So you can go jogging or walking while listening to music directly through your hearing aids. The future of hearing aid technology has never looked brighter. There are now common wireless standard and powerful low profile transmitters that hook into public address systems making public places such as auditoriums, theaters, airports, places of worship and even drive-up pharmacies and fast food restaurants accessible to people with hearing aids.[15] Be sure to explore Chapter 12 and Appendix I.

6. Controls on Your Hearing Aid

Your goal is to purchase a hearing aid that never needs adjustments. It should graciously determine the volume you need and adjust its directionality by sensing if you're in a quiet area or in a variety of noisy situations. A completely digital hearing aid, when it comes across steady state noise (like in an airplane cabin or around an air conditioner) should improve your hearing comfort in these situations by making the sounds more tolerable. In addition, it should not give you feedback as it amplifies sounds around you. It should restore your ability to enjoy some soft sounds (e.g., leaves rustling, bubbling of a fish tank, etc.) while sensing very loud sounds and making them comfortable for you (loud sounds should never be painful to your ears).

While the industry has in principle developed automatic hearing instruments, some people need to personally control them. Research has shown, especially among experienced wearers, that some people (roughly a third) still need either a volume control, multiple memory switch (quiet versus noisy situation switch), or a remote control in order to control volume or to access different hearing aid strategies for handling different listening environments. Some people need control of their hearing aid for the following reasons: the automatic feature does not meet their needs in 100 percent of listening situations; psychologically, these hearing aid wearers simply must have control of their hearing aids; or they are long-term hearing aid wearers habituated to a volume control and are therefore unwilling to part with it.

It's very important that you determine your needs with respect to control of the hearing aid. You don't want to fiddle with your hearing aids every ten minutes, but then again you don't want to be frustrated because your hearing aids work well in most situations, but not in ten percent of your favorite situations (e.g., listening to soft music). You need to explore this topic with your hearing health professional.

7. Sound Quality

One of the most important aspects of an enjoyable hearing aid experience is that you like the sound quality of hearing aids. So when you test-run your hearing aids, make sure that you consider the following dimensions of sound quality:

- Do you like the sound of your voice?
- Is the sound clean and crisp (sound clarity)?
- Is the sound too tinny?
- Are loud sounds uncomfortable to you?
- Does the world sound like you're in a barrel?
- Are your hearing aids natural sounding?
- Does it make some pleasant soft sounds audible to you?
- Does music sound pleasant and rich in texture?
- Does your hearing aid whistle, buzz, or squeal on its own?
- Does your hearing aid plug up your ears and muffle sound?

With today's modern digital hearing aids, most of these problems should be solved. If you notice any of these problems during the trial run and in your follow-up visits, by all means talk to your hearing healthcare professional about these issues. Such professionals are now capable of adjusting your hearing aids to your satisfaction. The extent to which all of the possible sound quality issues can be resolved, of course, depends on the severity of your hearing loss. In other words, some types of hearing losses are simply more conducive to restoration of rich sound quality in many listening environments while others are not.

8. Do Not Purchase Based Only on Cosmetics

Since the 1990s, the hearing aid industry has reduced the size of hearing aids to near invisibility especially with CICs and open fit hearing aids. Some people concerned with cosmetics prefer the least noticeable hearing aids, in the same way that they might choose contact lenses instead of framed eyeglasses. The problem is that the smallest hearing aid may not be the most suitable hearing solution for you for a variety of reasons. Your specific hearing loss may require more power than is available in CICs or open fit hearing aids.

Because of hearing loss stigma or embarrassment, many consumers come into hearing healthcare offices and start off the dialog with, "I would like one of those invisible hearing aids that I saw on TV." A likely response may be something like, "We carry invisible hearing aids, but I first need to examine your ears, measure your hearing loss, assess your lifestyle and manual dexterity, and then discuss how your hearing loss is impacting the quality of your life. You may or may not be a candidate for these invisible hearing aids." If it's determined that you're not a candidate, but you still insist on buying them, ethical hearing health providers will not fit you with the product because in essence they would be giving you the wrong prescription for your hearing loss.

9. Have Realistic Expectations during the Trial Period

The instructions you receive during the initial stages of adjustment are designed to help you formulate realistic expectations of what to expect from your hearing aids. You may need a specific wearing schedule for hearing aids. One experienced in-the-canal hearing aid wearer obtained CIC instruments a few years ago. He was in his early 30s and had used hearing aids since he was a teenager. When he returned for his recheck, he was asked how long he could wear the instruments in the beginning. He said that he could only use them for fifteen minutes at a time. Within two weeks, he was wearing them full-time, and they were completely comfortable. Had he not been counseled that adjusting to the deep insertion of the shell tip with CIC hearing aids may take extra time, he might have become discouraged and given up on that particular style of hearing aids.

Be patient with yourself. If you have the best hearing aids for your hearing loss and your lifestyle, hang in there. Make sure you're comfortable with the advice you've been given. Ask questions. Remember, your provider is your advocate. Satisfied hearing aid wearers are not shy when it comes to telling others about their success, but unfortunately, neither are the dissatisfied. No two people are alike, so don't assume if someone else has had a bad experience, all hearing aids are bad. You could very well be one of the overwhelming majority who has a good experience! There are many reasons why someone else may not have been successful, so don't project these conditions and improbabilities onto yourself. Also, do not expect someone else's hearing aids to work for you. Would you try on another person's eyeglasses and then decide whether you could be helped based on this experience?

Be realistic. Hearing aids will not permit you to hear the flapping of hummingbird wings over a lawnmower. Remember that it takes time to get used to hearing aids, especially if you're a new wearer. Keep in mind that background noise is almost always part of your environment, and adjustment to it is required. In time, you'll tune out many of these everyday sounds. It's important not to become disappointed or frustrated while your brain begins to adjust to a whole new world of sound. If you're an experienced wearer trying new hearing aids, understand that they might not sound like your old ones. Before you reject them, allow neural hook-ups in the auditory portion of the brain to adapt to these new sounds. You just might find that you like this new sound better than the old one.

Later on in this chapter I'll list what I've learned you should realistically expect from your hearing aids.

10. Earwax Protection

One of the common causes of hearing aid failure is moisture and earwax filling up the receiver tubing of the hearing aid, causing the speaker to malfunction. I strongly suggest that you take precaution to keep earwax out of the hearing aid. I've personally studied more than 90,000 hearing aid owners over a two-year period and determined that it's possible to reduce hearing aid repairs due to receiver failure by 50 percent by using a wax guard at the tip of the hearing aids.[16]

11. Counseling and Aural Rehabilitation

I would be oversimplifying the consumer journey with hearing aids if I stated that hearing loss rehabilitation involves only being fit with hearing aids. Some people with hearing loss will visit a hearing health professional, be tested, be fit with their hearing aids, and thereby derive optimal benefit. But many people, especially those who have delayed a solution for 20 years or who have more serious hearing losses, may need more help.

Less experienced hearing aid users should consider attending one-on-one or group sessions with their hearing health professional or doing independent study. If your hearing health professional does not offer aural rehabilitation (commonly comprising group discussion of hearing issues), by all means find a local group in your area that provides such training. A good starting point is to contact the Hearing Loss Association of America (www.hearingloss.org) to see if there's a self-help group in your area. The core of such training is well presented by Dr. Ross in Chapter 9. In addition, the Better Hearing Institute has provided a number of articles on the following topics (www.betterhearing.org under "Aural education and counseling"):

- resolution of any negative feelings you have about your hearing loss
- care and maintenance of your hearing aids
- communication strategies including assertiveness training, clear speech communication, and if necessary lipreading
- tips for hearing in noise
- your legal rights
- using computer software to retrain your brain to listen (e.g. LACE)
- the value of self-help groups
- airport screening tips

12. Assistive Listening Devices

For some people, especially those with severe hearing loss, hearing aids are not enough. Your hearing health professional will guide you through the array of technologies to further assist you to hear in the world. These devices may be FM hearing aids, companion microphones, Blue-tooth technology, telecoils for better hearing on the phone or for public places that are inductively looped, amplified telephones, specialized alarm clocks, and lamps that alert you better to your environment. If you have a telecoil in your hearing aid, by all means consider inductive looping your home so that you can hear your TV (and any other audio devices) directly into your hearing aids. (For more information on assistive listening technology, see Chapter 10, Appendix I, and visit www.betterhearing.org under "Hearing loss treatment/Assistive Listening Devices.")

Twelve Reasons to Purchase Two Hearing Aids Instead of One

Research with more than 5,000 consumers with hearing loss in both ears demonstrated that binaurally fit subjects (with two hearing aids) were more satisfied than those monaurally fit (with one hearing aid).[17-18] When given the choice and allowed to hear binaurally, the overwhelming majority of consumers (86 percent) chose two hearing aids over one.[1] Consequently, binaural users tend to communicate better in their place of worship, in small group gatherings, large gatherings, and even outdoors. Naturally, a person's ability to enjoy hearing aids will depend on the specific hearing loss and the type of technology used in the hearing aids.

Nevertheless, if you have a hearing loss in both ears and there is usable hearing in your poorer ear, budget permitting, I would recommend a hearing aid for both ears. Many hearing healthcare providers can demonstrate the binaural advantage on your very first visit, under headphone testing.

Based on a review of the literature and my own research with thousands of consumers with hearing loss in both ears, here are the reasons why you should consider a binaural hearing system when they're indicated.

1. Keeps both ears active, resulting in less hearing deterioration. As Dr. Carmen identifies in Chapter Two that research has shown that when only one hearing instrument is worn, the unaided ear tends to lose its ability to hear and understand. This is clinically called the *auditory deprivation effect.* People wearing two hearing instruments keep both ears active. In fact, wearing one hearing aid (when two are indicated) could result in greater deterioration of hearing in the unaided ear than if the person wore no hearing aid at all.

2. Better understanding of speech. Wearing two hearing instruments rather than one achieves selective listening more easily. Research shows that people wearing two hearing aids routinely understand speech and conversation significantly better than people wearing only one.

3. Better understanding in group and noisy situations. Wearing two hearing aids improves speech intelligibility in difficult listening situations. However, binaural digital technology tends to perform better in noise than older (analog) technologies.

4. Better ability to tell direction of sound. This is called localization. Research shows that in binaural use, there's an average of a 15 percent shift in increased satisfaction in "ability to tell the direction of sounds." This is a substantial improvement! In a social gathering, for example, localization allows you to hear from which direction someone is speaking to you. In traffic, you can tell from which direction a car or siren is coming.

5. Better sound quality. When you listen to a stereo system, you use both speakers to get the smoothest, sharpest, most natural sound quality. The same thing can be said of hearing aids. By wearing two hearing instruments, you increase your hearing range from 180 degrees reception (with just one instrument) to 360 degrees. This greater range provides a better sense of balance and sound quality.

6. Smoother tone quality. Wearing two hearing instruments generally requires less volume. This results in less distortion and more acceptable reproduction of sounds.

7. Reduced feedback and whistling. A lower volume control setting reduces the chances of feedback.

8. Wider hearing range. It's true. A person can hear sounds from a further distance with two ears, rather than just one. A voice that's barely heard at ten feet with one ear can be heard up to forty feet with two ears.

9. Better sound identification. Often, with just one hearing instrument, many noises and words sound alike. But with two hearing instruments, as with two ears, sounds are more easily distinguishable.

10. Hearing is less tiring and listening more pleasant. More binaural hearing aid wearers report that listening and participating in conversation are more enjoyable with two instruments. This is because you do not have to strain to hear with the better ear. Thus, binaural hearing can help make listening (and therefore life) more pleasant and relaxing.

11. Feeling of balanced hearing. Two-eared hearing results in a feeling of balanced reception of sound, also known as the stereo effect, whereas monaural hearing creates an unusual feeling of sounds being heard in one ear.

12. Tinnitus Masking. About 50 percent of people with ringing in their ears report improvement when wearing hearing aids. If you have a hearing aid in only one ear, there will still be ringing in the unaided ear.

How to Align Your Expectations with Hearing Aid Performance

Satisfaction with your hearing aids is highly dependent on the expectations you have. If you have unrealistic expectations, you'll be dissatisfied. Here are some issues you should keep in mind as you develop appropriate expectations about what your hearing aids can and <u>cannot</u> do for you.

- No matter how technically advanced, in most cases hearing aids cannot restore your hearing to normal except in some very mild hearing losses.
- Not all hearing aids perform the same with every type of hearing loss.
- No hearing aid will filter out all background noise. Some hearing instruments can reduce amplification of some types of background noise or make you more comfortable in the presence of noise.
- Where appropriate, directional microphones can often improve your ability to hear in noise.
- Directional hearing instruments coupled with digital signal processing will optimize your hearing instruments for improving your quality of life in noisy environments.
- Since you're purchasing custom hearing instruments, you should expect the fit to be comfortable; ideally you should not even know they're in your ears. There should not be any soreness, bleeding, or rashes associated with wearing hearing aids. If there is, go back to your hearing health provider to make adjustments to the shell of the aid or earmold.
- Hearing instruments should allow you to:
  (1) hear soft sounds (e.g., child's voice, soft speech) that you couldn't hear without amplification—this is part of the enjoyment of hearing aids;
  (2) understand speech in quiet situations—many people will derive some additional speech intelligibility in noise with advanced technology;
  (3) prevent loud sounds from becoming uncomfortably loud for you, but very loud sounds that are uncomfortable to normal hearing people may still be uncomfortable to you.

- Hearing aids may squeal or whistle when you're inserting them into your ear (if you don't have a volume control to shut it off); but if the aid squeals after the initial insertion, then most likely you have an inadequate fit and should tell your hearing health provider.
- Do not expect your friend's hearing aid brand or style to work for you.
- Do not expect your family doctor to know very much about hearing loss, brands of hearing aids, and your need for them.
- Expect your hearing aids to provide benefit to you during the trial period. By benefit, I mean that your ability to understand speech has demonstrably improved in the listening situations important to you (with realistic expectations though). This is what you paid for, so you should expect benefit. If you don't experience an improvement, then work with your hearing health professional to adjust the instrument to meet your specific needs. Never purchase a hearing aid that does not give you sufficient benefit.
- Expect to be satisfied with your hearing instruments and expect the quality of your life to improve.
- Expect a 30-day trial period with a money-back guarantee if your hearing aids do not give you benefit. (There might be a small nonrefundable portion for some services rendered.)
- Give your hearing aids a chance, being sure to follow the instructions of the hearing health provider. Most people need a period of adjustment (called acclimatization) before they're deriving maximum benefit (even up to four months).

Common Myths about Hearing Loss and Hearing Aids

There are many common myths still prevalent about hearing loss and hearing aids. I would like to dispel these myths now that you're living in the 21st Century.

"My hearing loss cannot be helped."

In the past, many people with hearing loss in one ear, with a high frequency hearing loss, or with nerve damage have all been told they cannot be helped, often by their family practice physician. This might have been true many years ago, but with modern advances in technology, the vast majority of people with a sensorineural hearing loss <u>can</u> benefit from hearing aids.

"Hearing loss affects only <u>old people</u> and is <u>a sign of aging</u>."

Only 40 percent of people with hearing loss are older than age 65. There are more than five million people in the U.S. between the ages of 18 and 44 with hearing loss, and more than one million are of school age. Hearing loss affects all age groups.

"If I had a hearing loss, my family doctor would have told me. "

Not true! Only 15 percent of physicians routinely screen for hearing loss during a physical. Since most hard of hearing people hear well in a quiet environment like your doctor's office, it can be virtually impossible for your physician to recognize the extent of your problem. Without special training in and understanding of the nature of hearing loss, it may be difficult for your doctor to even believe that you have a hearing problem.

Hearing aids will make me <u>look older</u> or <u>handicapped</u>."

Looking older is clearly more affected by almost all other factors besides hearing aids. It's not the hearing aids that make one look older, it's the way you conduct yourself in the absence of hearing aids. If hearing aids help you function like a normal hearing person, for all intents and purposes, the stigma is removed. Hearing aid manufacturers are well aware that cosmetics are an issue to many people, and that's why today we have hearing aids that fit totally in the ear canal (essentially not noticeable unless someone is staring directly into your ear). These CIC and open fit styles of hearing aids have enough power and special features to satisfy at least half of individuals with hearing loss. Smiling and nodding your head when you don't understand what's being said make your condition more apparent than the largest hearing aid.

"The consequences of hiding hearing loss are better than wearing hearing aids."

What price are you paying for vanity? I go back to the old adage that an untreated hearing loss is far more noticeable than hearing aids. If you miss a punch line to a joke or respond inappropriately in conversation, people may have concerns about your mental acuity, your attention span, or your ability to communicate effectively. The personal consequences of vanity can be life altering. At a simplistic level, untreated hearing loss means giving up some of the pleasant sounds you used to enjoy. At a deeper level, vanity could severely reduce the quality of your life.

"Only people with serious hearing loss need hearing aids."

The need for hearing amplification is dependent on your lifestyle, your need for refined hearing, and the degree of your hearing loss. If you're a lawyer, teacher, or a group psychotherapist, where very acute hearing is necessary to discern the nuances of human communication, then even a mild hearing loss can be unacceptable. If you live in a rural area by yourself and seldom socialize, then perhaps you're someone who can disregard treatment.

"I'll just have some minor surgery like my friend did, and then my hearing will be okay."

Many people know someone whose hearing improved after medical or surgical treatment, and it's true that some types of hearing loss can be successfully treated. With adults, unfortunately, this only applies to five to ten percent of cases, and is most often associated with ear infections.

"My hearing loss is normal for my age."

Isn't this a strange way to look at things? But, do you realize that well-meaning physicians tell this to their patients every day? It happens to be "normal" for overweight people to have high blood pressure or diabetes. That doesn't mean they should not receive treatment for the problem.

"I have one ear that's down a little, but the other one's okay."

Everything is relative. Nearly all patients with bilateral hearing loss believe they have <u>one good ear</u>, but they actually have <u>two bad ears</u>. When one ear is slightly better than the other, we learn to favor that ear for the telephone, group conversations, and so forth. It can give the illusion that "the better ear" is normal. Most types of hearing loss affect both ears fairly equally, and about 90 percent of patients with bilateral hearing loss are in need of hearing aids for both ears.

"Hearing aids will make everything sound too loud."

Hearing aids are amplifiers. At one time, the way hearing aids were designed, it was necessary to turn up the power in order to hear soft speech (or other soft sounds). With today's digital technology hearing aids, the circuit works automatically, only providing the amplification needed based on the input level. In fact, many hearing aids today don't have a volume control.

Conclusions

Hopefully, you now recognize the value of hearing aids and the significant impact they can have on your life, as well as the life of your family, loved ones and associates. I also hope you realize that hearing aids may not necessarily be an instant cure for your hearing difficulties, but with patience, you'll find they can be your bridge to healing.

References

1. Kochkin S. (2009). MarkeTrak VIII: 25 year trends in the hearing health market. *The Hearing Review*, 16 (11): 12-31.

2. Kochkin S, Tyler, R. & Born J. (2011). MarkeTrak VIII: Prevalence of Tinnitus and Efficacy of Treatments, *The Hearing Review*, 18 (12): 10-26

3. Kochkin S. (2000). MarkeTrak V: Why my hearing aids are in the drawer: the consumer's perspective. *The Hearing Journal*, 53 (2): 34-42.

4. Kochkin S. (2007). MarkeTrak VII: Obstacles to adult non-user adoption of hearing aids. *The Hearing Journal*, 60 (4): 27-43.

5. Kochkin S. (2012). MarkeTrak VIII: The key influencing factors in hearing aid purchase intent. *The Hearing Review*, 19 (3):12-25.

6. Kochkin S. (2010). MarkeTrak VIII: Customer satisfaction with hearing aids is slowly increasing. *The Hearing Journal*, 63 (1): 11-19.

7. Kochkin S. (2011). MarkeTrak VIII: Patients report improved quality of life with hearing aid usage, *The Hearing Journal*, Vol. 64 (6): 25-32.

8. Kochkin S. (2011). MarkeTrak VIII: Mini-BTEs tap new market, users more satisfied, *The Hearing Journal*, 64 (3): 17-18, 20, 22, 24.

9. Kochkin S. (2000). Customer satisfaction with single and multiple microphone digital hearing aids, *The Hearing Review*, 7 (11): 24-29.

10. Kochkin S. (2005). MarkeTrak VII: Customer Satisfaction with Hearing Aids in the Digital Age, *The Hearing Journal*, 58 (9): 30-37.

11. Kochkin S & Rogin C. (2000). Quantifying the obvious: the impact of hearing aids on quality of life, *The Hearing Review*, 7 (1): 8-34.

12. Singer J, Healey J & Preece J. (1997). Hearing instruments: a psychological and behavioral perspective. *High Performance Hearing Solutions* 1: 23-27.

13. Kochkin S. (2005). Customer satisfaction with hearing aids in the Digital Age. *The Hearing Journal*, 58 (9): 30-37.

14. Kochkin S. (1996). Customer satisfaction and subjective benefit with high-performance hearing instruments. *The Hearing Review*, 3(12): 16-26.

15. Kochkin S. (2007). Increasing hearing aid adoption through multiple environmental listening utility. *The Hearing Journal,* 60 (11), 28-49.

16. Kochkin S. (2002). Finally a solution to the cerumen problem. *The Hearing Review*, 9 (4): 46-49.

17. Kochkin S & Kuk F. (1997). The binaural advantage: evidence from subjective benefit and customer satisfaction data. *The Hearing Review*, 4 (4): 29, 30-32, 34.

18. Kochkin S. (2000). Binaural hearing aids: the fitting of choice for bilateral loss subjects. Itasca, IL: Knowles Electronics, Retrieved from the Better Hearing Institute: http://www.betterhearing.org/pdfs/Binaural_hearing_aid_complete_review.pdf.

19. Allen R. (2002). Reasonable expectations for the consumer. Retrieved from www.healthyhearing.com.

20. Stypulkowski P. (1997). Realistic expectations: a key to success. *High Performance Hearing Solutions,* 1: 56-57.

CHAPTER EIGHT
Mapping Your Audiogram
Kris English, PhD

Dr. English earned her PhD at San Diego State University and Claremont Graduate University. She is a professor at the University of Akron, She has authored numerous books, chapters and papers, most lately addressing the adjustment process to living with hearing loss. She is active with the American Academy of Audiology, haing served as President in 2009-2010. She and her husband live in constant amazement that their two children are now adults and managing life on their own just fine.

Understanding how to read your own audiogram will assist you in better understanding your personal hearing challenges. As with anything new, it will seem a little complicated, so this chapter breaks down its components for easier understanding. In my discussion with you, I will present "Mini-Summaries" of each section, provided throughout to review vocabulary and concepts, and occasionally "Audiogram Alerts" are provided to highlight a particular point of concern. In time, you will be an expert in describing your audiogram. Obtain a copy of your audiogram before reading this chapter, so we can work together in this exploration. You'll have the opportunity to fill in the graph in Figure 8-1 with your audiogram once we get through enough of this chapter for you to understand what you'll see.

An audiogram has three main components:
1. A range of pitches, from low to high.
2. A measurement of loudness, from soft to very loud.
3. Your hearing levels for each pitch for each ear.

Audiogram Components

Audiogram Component #1: Pitch
The first component of the audiogram is the range of pitches presented in the hearing test. Wearing headphones or insert earphones, you heard a series of beeps that may have reminded you of notes on a piano. Some had very low pitches (like the deep bass notes on the left end of the piano keys), some were very high pitches (similar to the far right end of piano keys), and some were in

between. These pitches are lined up on the horizontal part of the audiogram, as shown in Figure 8-1.

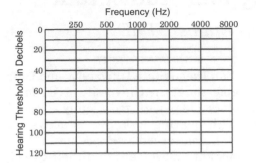

Figure 8-1: pitch and loudness on an audiogram

Another term used to describe these beeps is "pure tones." You may have noticed each beep was like a single note on a piano, with no chords or harmonics. The human ear can hear pure tones much lower and higher than the ones shown on the audiogram, but it would take too much time to test them all. For efficiency's sake we focus on what people are most interested in hearing—human speech. So the pure tones found in human speech are selected for testing and are the ones reported on your audiogram.

It may seem a little strange to say these pure tones have anything to do with human speech, but when analyzed electronically, each speech sound has been found to be a unique and complex combination of these pure tones. That's why your hearing care professional started with pure tone testing, as a way to describe the "building blocks" of your hearing ability.

Chances are, the term "frequency" was used during an explanation of your hearing test. For example, you may have been told you have a "high frequency hearing loss." Frequency means *pitch*: it refers to the number of cycles a sound wave occurs in one second. A sound that vibrates your eardrum at 500 times or cycles per second (cps) is perceived by your brain as having a low pitch, like the hum of the motor in your refrigerator. As the vibrations per second increase, the pitch of the sound will seem higher and higher, like the cheep of a bird.

A scientist named Heinrich Hertz (1857-1894) described this idea of low and high pitches having different cycles per second, and in his honor, his initials are now used to replace *cps* with *Hz*. So, for example, your hearing test may indicate that you have a hearing loss at 8000 Hz. Because this pitch (frequency) occurs in the higher end of the area for speech sounds, it can also be said to be a high frequency hearing loss.

Mini-Summary

All of these terms mean the same thing:
- A high frequency hearing loss
- A hearing loss in the higher pitches
- A hearing loss at 4000-8000 Hz

Audiogram Component #2: Loudness

The first question we want to answer is: how loud does each pitch have to be for you to hear it? Loudness is recorded on the vertical part of the audiogram (Figure 8-1). The unit of measure for loudness is the decibel (abbreviated dB). The audiogram uses increments of 5 dB mainly because the human ear is not usually able to notice differences of less than 5 dB.

This vertical measurement often causes some confusion. The softest levels of hearing are at the top, so the loudness *increases* as it goes *down* the scale. Initially, it might seem more logical to place the softest levels on the bottom and then, as loudness goes up, the scale should go up. So watch for this, and remember: when the loudness of the pitch needs to be increased, it means the hearing level is dropping downward.

Mini-Summary

- Pitch or frequency is measured in Hertz (Hz).
- Loudness is measured in decibels (dB).
- These two measures are combined to tell us how loud (in dB) you need each frequency (Hz) to be in order to just barely hear it. This is called your *hearing threshold* for that frequency, and will be explained further in the next section.

Audiogram Component #3: Your Hearing in Each Ear

Hearing tests usually start with the middle pitch, 1000 Hz. Let's say your right ear is being tested first. The tester sets the equipment to this frequency, and you raise your finger or push a button every time you hear it. The pure tone gets softer and softer, until you can barely perceive it. That level is your *threshold* for that frequency. Threshold means the softest level you could perceive it.

If your threshold in the right ear for 1000 Hz is 30 dB, the tester records it with a circle at the intersection of those two values (Figure 8-2). Another threshold is then obtained at 2000 Hz, in this example, 40 dB. This procedure is repeated for each frequency. Then the other ear is tested in the same way.

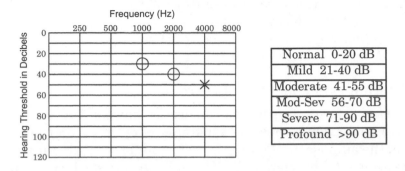

Figure 8-2: three thresholds

In Figure 8-2, the "X" found at 45 dB at 4000 Hz represents a threshold for the left ear. How will you remember which symbol is for which ear? The letter *R* will keep things straight: the *right* ear uses a *round* symbol (the circle). And if the hearing care professional used headphones to test your hearing, the *red* headphone went on your *right* ear. It's easy to remember because the "R" is the first letter in **r**ed, **r**ight and **r**ound—*aha!* Once you know the "round" symbols describe the right ear's hearing levels, by default you know the "X" stands for left ear hearing levels.

You may have had your hearing tested not only with headphones or inserts, but also with a bone oscillator that typically rested on your mastoid bone (behind your ear on the skull). The hearing information obtained with the oscillator would be reported with carats (^ or < or >) or brackets. They are not included here in our first few audiograms in order to make this a bit more user-friendly; however, an example will be seen later (Figure 8-9).

Mini-Summary

- Each pitch is tested to see how loud it needs to be for you to just barely hear it. This is your threshold for each pitch.
- The hearing levels for the right ear are depicted with Os, and the left ear is depicted with Xs.

🎦 Audiogram Alert!

On any given day, a person's hearing levels for pure tones can go up or down by about 5 dB. For example, on Monday a threshold at 1000 Hz could be 35; on Tuesday it could be 30, and on Wednesday it could be 40. This 5 dB variability is normal, and can be explained by a variety of reasons. For example, if you're fatigued, your threshold could go down 5 dB because it takes a lot of concentration to keep listening to very soft tones. There's also evidence that diet plays a role in hearing. For example, the ear depends on a delicate balance of salt and potassium. If these levels are thrown off, hearing can be affected.

While a 5 dB variability is not a concern, keep an eye on your first (baseline) hearing test. From one year to the next, a 5 dB shift might not seem unusual, but a 5 dB downward shift every year will have an impact on what hearing aids are selected for you.

"Give it to Me Straight, Doc—How Bad is My Hearing?"

Figure 8-3 shows our three audiogram components with a complete pure tone hearing test. The Os and Xs are connected with lines to help the eye track the hearing levels across the pitches. But what does it all mean? This takes us to the next step in interpreting your audiogram.

Hearing levels can be described in a progression of loss: normal, mild, moderate, moderately severe, severe, or profound. These levels of loss are added to Figure 8-3. The hearing levels depicted here are typical for many patients. Both ears start off at normal levels in the low pitches, drop to a mild loss in the middle pitches, and then end with a moderate loss in the high pitches.

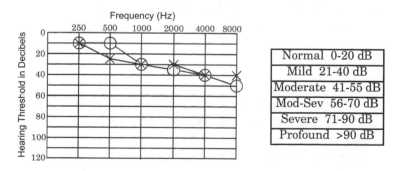

Figure 8-3: mild to moderate hearing loss both ears

Because there are different hearing levels (normal and also mild and moderate degrees of hearing loss) across the pitches, how would you describe this hearing loss?

Your hearing report would probably reveal close to what is written in the previous paragraph, but in conversation, you can accurately say this person has a mild to moderate hearing loss in the mid to high frequencies, both ears.

Figure 8-4 demonstrates how as the loudness increases, the hearing levels drop down the audiogram. In this example, the hearing loss we saw in Figure 8-3 has dropped about 10 to 45 dB, indicating moderate-to-severe hearing loss in both ears.

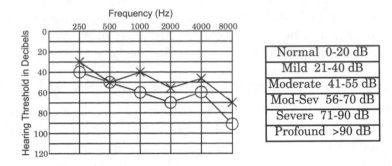

Figure 8-4: moderate to severe hearing loss both ears

By the way, in this chapter I am assuming that you're experiencing a hearing loss in both ears (called a bilateral loss). Occasionally, individuals have hearing loss only in one ear, with normal hearing in the other. This condition is called a unilateral (one-sided) hearing loss, and it presents unique challenges in localizing sound sources and listening in noise. Ask your hearing health professional for more information if you have a unilateral hearing loss.

Mini-Summary

- Hearing levels can be summarized with descriptors such as normal, mild, moderate, moderately severe, severe, and profound.
- These descriptors may need to be combined to describe all the pitches (from low, middle, and high) accurately.
- How you hear pure tones is directly related to how you hear

speech—the ultimate question you want to answer. Your test may have included how soft you could hear speech (speech recognition threshold, reported in decibels). These results are often included on the same form as your audiogram.

⊞ Audiogram Alert!

Occasionally, you will hear people use percentages to describe their hearing loss, as in "I was told I have a 50 percent loss in my right ear." There are two circumstances that could explain this kind of description. First, the American Medical Association developed a percentage system years ago to describe hearing loss, and occasionally physicians still use it. However, as you look at an audiogram, you can see that decibels do not translate into percentages, and the hearing levels for each pitch are not addressed at all. So the percentage system, while intending to be helpful, does not really tell you much, and could even be misleading.

The other explanation could be a confusion with some audiological testing that *is* reported in percentages. In addition to finding out how you heard pure tones, your hearing care professional may have also wanted to know how well you hear one-syllable words. This is necessary to understand your hearing difficulties, and will be touched on in Dr. Sandlin's chapter.

The Connection from Pure Tones to Speech Sounds

All along I have been saying that the pure tones by which you had been tested are related to how you hear and understand speech. Figure 8-5 (next page) is an audiogram with speech sounds superimposed over it. It shows how speech sounds are spread out in pitch. It's been noted that this shape vaguely resembles a banana, so it is often called the "speech banana."

Vowels are relatively low in pitch, while consonants that use voicing (for example, /l/, /m/, /n/) are in the middle range of pitches. "Voicing" means your voice helps produce the sound. To experience this, place your finger tips on your throat and hum a long "mmm." You'll feel your throat vibrate. You're feeling your larynx (voice box) move as air travels from your lungs to your mouth.

Many speech sounds are high in pitch (for example, /s/ and /f/). These are produced without voicing, making them extremely soft as well as high-pitched. For example, put your upper teeth over your lower lip and gently blow through. This is the position for /f/. Without using your voice, try to blow harder, attempting to make the /f/ sound louder. You'll immediately notice that it cannot be done very well because the power for speech comes from your voice. The /f/ is voiceless. Now add your voice to it by humming through your lips in the same position. By doing this, you now no longer have an /f/ but a /v/ because you added vocalization, which will make this sound *much* easier to hear.

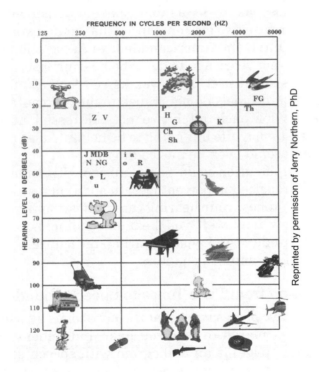

Figure 8-5: "Familiar Sounds" audiogram

All sounds for speech vibrate at different frequencies, which is how you differentiate speech sounds. Two of the highest consonant sounds in English are /f/ and /s/. Even a mild hearing loss in the high frequencies can make either sound inaudible. If you miss hearing only one sound in one word in a single sentence, it can be enough to misunderstand the entire message. This is also why some sounds seem garbled or muffled. It may sound like someone is mumbling. This situation explains the observation made by many people with hearing loss: "I can hear you, I just can't understand you!" Not picking up some of the speech sounds will make speech difficult to understand, although general speech activity can still be heard.

As hearing levels drop, more and more speech sounds become harder to hear. This is the information your hearing care professional is looking to assess in order to appropriately fit you with hearing aids, but it all starts with those pure tones.

⊞ Audiogram Alert!

Your hearing care professional may have spent some time explaining your audiogram to you once the testing was completed. If you found it confusing, you may have felt too distracted or overwhelmed with the confirmation of having a hearing loss. Don't be discouraged! It's a lot of information to take in, and you should give yourself credit for getting this far in this chapter.

More Practice

The more audiograms you see, the more sense they make. Following are four additional audiograms to consider before we take a look at your own audiogram. Figure 8-6 shows normal hearing in both ears up to 2000 Hz. Hearing levels drop to a moderate loss at 4000 Hz, and then recover to a mild loss at 8000 Hz. This type of configuration usually suggests a history of excessive noise exposure. It's such a commonly observed configuration, it has its own name: "noise notch." A person with this kind of hearing loss is strongly advised to take every measure necessary to protect against further noise exposure. Without hearing protection, this hearing loss can drop more and more, and eventually affect the middle and high frequencies.

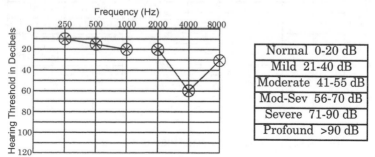

Figure 8-6: hearing loss consistent with noise exposure

Many hearing losses show gradual change from one frequency to the next, but some people have the kind of hearing loss shown in

Figure 8-7. We see normal hearing in both ears through 1000 Hz, and then a dramatic, precipitous drop at 2000 Hz. Typically, 1500 Hz is not tested but because of the difference between 1000 and 2000, this information is important to collect. This audiogram represents a moderately severe to profound hearing loss in the mid to high frequencies, right ear worse than left.

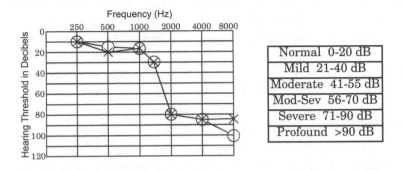

Figure 8-7: normal hearing in low pitches with a severe precipitous drop

In comparison, Figure 8-8 shows a severe-to-profound hearing loss in all the speech frequencies. No speech sounds produced at normal volume will be audible, although loud sounds in the environment might be barely heard.

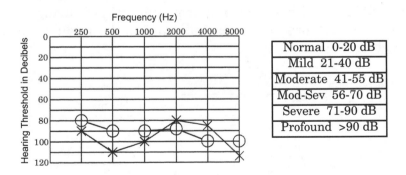

Figure 8-8: severe to profound hearing loss both ears

If you're a typical person with hearing loss, you have a sensorineural type of loss, meaning the sensory organ of hearing (the inner ear) is permanently losing its sensitivity. But hearing can also be temporarily affected by middle ear problems. These changes could be caused by severe head colds, allergies, damaged eardrums or other medical problems. This kind of hearing problem (called a conductive loss) will also be reflected in the audiogram, and we have one example here.

Looking only at the Os and Xs, Figure 8-9 indicates that a severe hearing loss exists in both ears in the low frequencies, recovering to a moderate hearing loss in the middle and high frequencies. However, when listening to pure tones with a bone oscillator (shown with bracket symbols), this person has better hearing levels in the low frequencies than indicated with headphones alone. Because of a middle ear problem, it's even harder than usual to hear low frequencies (note the poorer hearing levels). When a conductive loss is combined with a sensorineural loss, it's described as a *mixed loss*. Middle ear problems usually can be treated with medications or surgery. A person with an audiogram like one in Figure 8-9 will have better hearing if the conductive components are resolved (although a moderate sensorineural loss will remain in those lower frequencies).

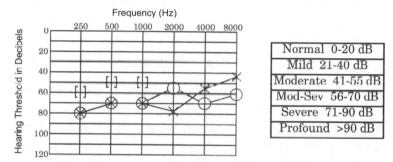

Figure 8-9: moderate sensorineural hearing loss both ears, with additional middle ear (conductive) hearing loss in lower frequencies

We've already briefly discussed Figures 8-6 through 8-9, so let's consider the remaining audiograms. If you have a hearing loss of some degree in the low and perhaps middle frequencies, and normal hearing in the higher ranges, this kind of hearing loss is often caused by health conditions such as diabetes, Ménière's disease, or labyrinthitis (see Chapter Seven, Q&A#9). This suggests that you might have some concomitant issues such as dizziness, vertigo, tinnitus or nausea. You could be missing as much as 30 percent of speech information, and like all hearing loss configurations, you probably find it hard to understand people in noisy situations. In this case, your audiogram will closely resemble Figure 8-10. Hearing aids will help you hear better.

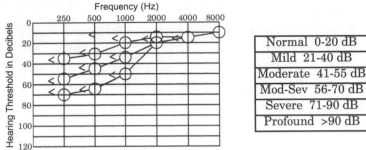

Figure 8-10: a variety of low frequency sensorineural hearing losses right ear only

Keep in mind that the more normal your hearing across the frequency ranges, especially progressing into the higher ranges, the better you'll function in your hearing world.

If your audiogram closely resembles Figures 8-11, 8-12 or 8-13, you have a mild hearing loss. You could be missing up to 40% of speech, making it difficult to follow conversations, especially in noisy situations (restaurants, parties, meetings). With these kinds of hearing losses, it isn't unusual for you to hear perfectly in some situations while struggling in others. This is the unpredict-able nature of living with mild sensorineural hearing loss. It can make you (and your family, friends and co-workers) wonder if you even have a hearing loss. Don't let it fool you or the family. It will almost always come down to the environment: too much background noise, too far away from the speaker, or someone isn't speaking loud enough.

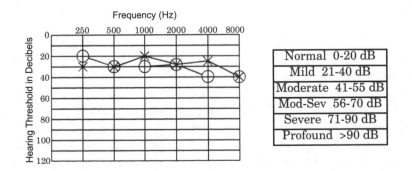

Figure 8-11: mild hearing loss both ears all frequencies (flat mild loss)

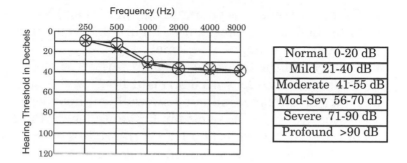

Figure 8-12: mild mid-to-high frequency hearing loss both ears (with normal hearing in lows)

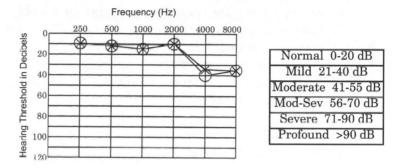

Figure 8-13: normal hearing low and mid frequencies with a mild loss in the high frequencies

You'll note that Figures 8-12 and 8-13 have hearing loss restricted to only the higher ranges. Figure 8-13 is limited to loss only in the uppermost range (furthest to the right on the audiogram). The latter indicates that someone with this loss may hear fairly well overall except when in the most challenging situations around noise or very soft female voices, and may not be the best candidate for hearing aids. Persons with audiograms similar to Figures 8-11 and 8-12 might well utilize hearing aids requiring only a minimum of power to pick up softer consonants that make speech clearer.

Now it's Your Turn!

To help translate this chapter into personally meaningful information, the following questions are presented. Please locate a copy of your audiogram and follow these easy steps:

1. Carefully transcribe your audiogram's Os and Xs in pencil onto the blank audiogram in Figure 3-1 (you can always erase it if it changes over time)
2. Connect all the Os with a straight line.
3. Connect all the Xs with a straight line.
4. Now you want to find out how well you hear within the critical range of hearing for human speech. Find your hearing threshold at 500 Hz for the right ear by looking on the graph below 500 until you see the O.
5. What is the dB level? Write it in here: _____ dB.
6. Look at the notation to the right that reveals the range from *normal* to *profound*, and write what yours is: _____.
7. Do the same for 4000 Hz as you just did for 500 Hz.
8. What is the range from *normal* to *profound* for 4000 Hz? Write what yours is: _____.
9. What are the ranges where your hearing levels start and end (for example, "*moderate* to *severe*" or perhaps even "*mild*" across all frequencies)? _____.
10. For the right ear, you should now know the range of loss you have. You can now do the same for the left ear.
11. Left ear loss at 500 Hz is: _____.
12. Left ear loss at 4000 Hz is: _____.
13. Left ear range of loss at 500 Hz is: _____.
14. Left ear range of loss at 4000 Hz is: _____.
15. What is the final range of hearing for your left ear (for example, *mild* to *severe*)? _____.
16. Now locate one of the many audiograms among Figures 3-6 through 3-20 in this chapter that most resembles your own audiogram. An easy way to match this is by noting your hearing levels for one ear at a time. Observe your loss only at these four frequencies: 500, 1000, 2000 and 4000 Hz and determine the best match for one ear.
17. You can now read the interpretation for the audiogram you matched, as described in that Figure. Ask yourself, what speech sounds are you missing? (see Figure 3-5 to find the answer to this question.) Are you a hearing aid candidate? What challenges lie ahead for you?
18. Repeat the match for the other ear if the hearing levels differ from the first ear's best match.

If your audiogram closely resembles Figures 8-14, 8-15 or 8-16, you have a moderate hearing loss at some of the tested frequencies. However, depending on where your loss occurs in the frequency range, you'll experience a different set of problems. Naturally, the further away you are from the conversation you are trying to hear, the more difficult it'll be for you to understand.

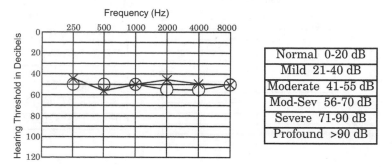

Figure 8-14: moderate hearing loss in all frequencies (moderate flat loss) both ears

Figure 8-14 indicates that with about equal loss across all tested frequencies, understanding almost all speech at five feet in a quiet room could prove challenging. For example, if a friend or family member was reading out loud behind a newspaper, yet only five feet away, you will not have the advantage of lipreading and would likely miss most of what was said.

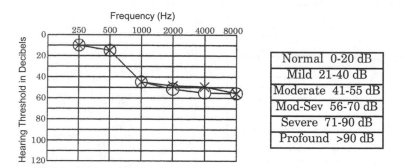

Figure 8-15: moderate mid-to-high frequency hearing loss both ears with normal hearing in the lows

On the other hand, if your loss is limited to only the high range, you'll likely to do much better. As you have no doubt already noticed, noisy situations make hearing even more difficult. Many of these environmental intrusions you can control yourself, such as turning down the music or television. Hearing aids are especially helpful with these kinds of hearing losses, shown in Figure 8-16, since they greatly assist in bringing back the intelligibility of speech.

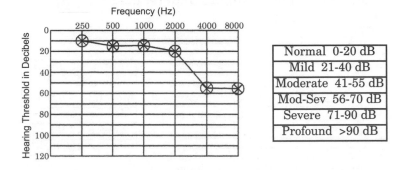

Figure 8-16: normal hearing in low and mid frequencies, with a moderate loss in the high frequencies for both ears

If your audiogram closely resembles Figure 8-17, you have a severe hearing loss across all frequencies. You already know that speech is not audible to you, and that hearing aids must be used in order to hear people and the sounds in your environment. The better your word discrimination ability under sound booth testing conditions without hearing aids, the better your prognosis for benefit with hearing aids in the "outside world."

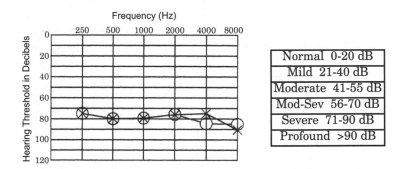

Figure 8-17: severe hearing loss in all frequencies both ears

If you are someone who has spent a career around toxic levels of noise (compressors, hammers, drills, saws, etc.), your audiogram resembles Figure 8-18. You are hearing mostly vowels—lots of vocal energy with not much clarity. The intelligibility for speech (consonants) is at best very muffled. You're missing a considerable percentage of conversation and your use of hearing aids is both necessary and probably beneficial, especially if your word recognition ability was tested and found to be good.

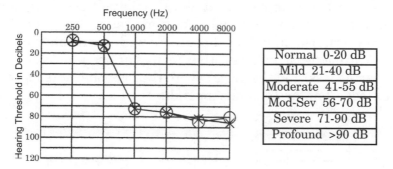

Figure 8-18: severe mid-to-high frequency hearing loss both ears with normal low frequencies

Figure 8-19 indicates normal hearing levels in the low-mid range, but severe high frequency loss. This audiogram includes testing at 3000 Hz, showing a more accurate picture of your hearing and potential challenges. High frequency consonants will be very difficult to hear (such as /f/, /k/, /s/ or /th/) and in the presence of some background noise, missed entirely. This audiogram typifies those with extensive firearms exposure. Hearing aids provide emphasis to the high frequencies and can fill in much of what you're missing.

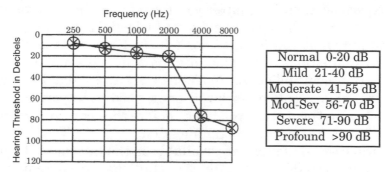

Figure 8-19: normal hearing in mid and low frequencies with a severe hearing loss in the high frequencies both ears

If your audiogram resembles Figure 8-20, you're already aware that you experience a profound loss in all frequencies. Powerful hearing aids are probably something you've been wearing for some time in order to receive as much auditory information as possible from speech and environmental sounds. If you're new to hearing aids with this kind of loss, you might consider exploring other options, such as a cochlear implant or a wide variety of assistive devices. Implants are increasingly viable options for many patients, but candidacy criteria must be discussed with your physician and hearing care professional. Assistive devices are helpful to all persons with hearing loss, and the more severe the loss, the more helpful the devices (see Chapter Ten and Appendix I).

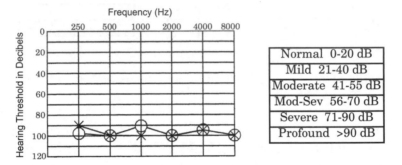

Figure 8-20: profound hearing loss in all frequencies both ears

A Demonstration Might Help Your Loved Ones

The audiogram is an abstract representation that provides important information to hearing care professionals. You've been working through a learning process to translate that information to your experiences, but no matter what kind of audiogram you have, it won't mean much to your family and friends. For other people to understand what you hear, or don't hear, I recommend that they listen to simulations of hearing loss, particularly simulations that recreate your own audiogram. You're already aware that hearing loss is an invisible problem, so loved ones need to experience it for themselves, or "hear what you hear," before they can empathize and work with you to improve communication.

Several free simulations are available on the Internet to help your family and friends appreciate the challenge of listening with diminished hearing. Using a search engine such as Google, type in "simulated hearing loss" or "hearing loss simulation" to find these helpful websites. At the time of this writing, the following websites are available and highly recommended:

- Better Hearing Institute
  http://www.betterhearing.org/sound
- National Institute for Health and Safety (NIOSH)
  http://www.cdc.gov/niosh/mining/content/hlsoundslike.html
- University of Wisconsin – Whitewater
  http://facstaff.uww.edu/bradleys/radio/hlsimulation

You may find it very helpful to ask family members or friends to discuss what they heard in the simulations, and also their reactions to hearing speech that is too soft, or distorted and muffled. They'll likely describe a need to increase concentration, a sense of frustration and then an inclination to "tune out" when the effort became too burdensome. These insights can lead to recalling times when they thought you were ignoring them. The extra effort needed to listen with hearing loss is also invisible, so it needs to be discussed for others to understand your challenge.

Audiograms are Not the Whole Story

We've spent considerable time reviewing how hearing levels are objectively measured and recorded. One final point must be mentioned: an audiogram does not always predict how you experience life. As you'll note throughout this book, two people can have identical audiograms but have very different reactions to the stresses and problems hearing loss causes. One person with mild to moderate hearing loss may experience a great deal of difficulty while another person with the same hearing loss (or worse) may have fewer challenges. Why would this be?

It seems to boil down to our individuality—the uniqueness that identifies each of us for who we are: our personality type, our perception of ourselves, our view of the world, and even our desire or motivation to communicate. A housebound reclusive person may be less likely to pursue hearing aids than an extraverted individual who continually engages with people to experience the joys of life. The truth is, as Dr. Carmen presented in the second chapter, some people have just grown accustomed to, and feel safer, living in their own world of untreated hearing loss while others are driven to solve their hearing problem.

Your hearing care professional would not assume that by knowing your audiogram, he or she also knows your listening challenges. Let your practitioner know your hearing needs and expectations so you can receive the maximum benefit with the technology now available to you. Help fill in the information that the audiogram cannot: your challenges with phone use, conferences at work, television at home, following sporting or musical events, and so on. Your audiogram provides the foundation for a personalized rehabilitation plan; building the actual plan is a team effort.

CHAPTER NINE

Improving Your Listening And Hearing Skills

Mark Ross, PhD

Dr. Ross received his doctorate at Stanford University. He has worked as a clinical audiologist, a director of a school for the deaf, Director of Research and Training at the League for the Hard of Hearing, and as a Professor of Audiology at the University of Connecticut where he's now a Professor Emeritus. Dr. Ross writes from his experience of someone who has personally worn hearing devices for over 60 years, ranging from vacuum tube body worn hearing aids to cochlear implants.

I don't know any hard of hearing person who, if a magic wand were available to wave away his or her hearing loss, would not jump at this miraculous opportunity. I know that I would like to be at the head of the line! But life is not a fairy tale and magic wands are in short supply. For most of us with hearing loss, it's simply a pain, one whose impact we're constantly trying to overcome or minimize.

We don't approach the world as hard of hearing people, seeking acceptance as a separate social entity. On the contrary, we're trying not to make the hearing loss the defining element of our personal identity; we do this, not by ignoring it, but by striving to reduce its impact in our lives. To realize our goal of continued engagement with the larger society—with our friends, family, jobs, and interests—we employ all the technological tools we can, i.e., hearing aids and other hearing assistive devices. And we use various communication strategies to reduce the inevitable consequences of hearing loss.

By *communication strategies* I mean any activity that might increase your ability to understand speech, either generally or in particular situations, not just technological solutions. Of course technology is a key consideration, but the adjustment process doesn't end there. There are other things you can do to improve your ability to communicate in different situations. When you purchase hearing instruments, you depend upon the hearing healthcare provider's expertise to help in making the proper decision. When it comes to communication strategies and making the best use of all types of hearing technology, you have to take the major responsibility. The concept of personal responsibility for your own action underlies the three recurring themes stressed throughout this chapter: acknowledgment, assertiveness, and communication strategies.

I'll begin this chapter by discussing your personal responsibilities as you strive to improve your hearing capabilities, after which I'll comment on your initial experiences with hearing aids. My focus will be on how you can learn to interpret, enjoy and expand the new world of sound to which you've suddenly been exposed. I'll follow this by discussing speechreading and auditory training exercises that can help you make the most of your residual hearing. Finally, in the last section, I'll present some *hearing tactics*, i.e., various kinds of adaptations to real-life situations aimed at improving speech comprehension. In writing this chapter, I've drawn heavily on what I've personally practiced during the many years that I've worn hearing aids (and I shudder to think what my life would have been be like without them).

Acknowledgment

The first and indispensable step in practicing effective communication strategies is to accept the reality of the hearing loss. Unless and until you can acknowledge its presence, openly and in a matter of fact way, you're always going to be limited in how effectively you can deal with it. A hearing loss is not something to be ashamed of; it's not a stigma that has to be hidden. Its presence does not diminish you as a human being. By denying or projecting your hearing difficulties onto other people's mouths ("People don't talk as clearly as they used to!"), you fool only yourself. The point is worth emphasizing. The hearing loss is there. Magical thinking, denial, not wanting to talk about it will not make it go away. If you don't face up to this reality, unpleasant as it may be, you may be condemning yourself to a life of unnecessary stress, anxiety and isolation. If you've read the previous chapters by Dr. Carmen and Dr. Kochkin, you know this is true.

The onset of a hearing loss is typically very gradual. What makes this situation particularly difficult for older people is that, initially, they're truly not aware that a hearing loss may be the main reason they're having communication difficulties. They can't very well deny hearing sounds to which they're unaware! This is the point where many of the conflicts between the hard of hearing person and his/her significant others first arise. It's not so much denial as disbelief; they know there are times when they can hear well. After a while, of course, the effects of the hearing loss become apparent to everyone, including the person involved. If these are ignored, then someone can truly be said to be "in denial." And since older people are also more likely to exhibit behavioral symptoms of dementia it may be tempting to dismiss the hearing loss effects as those caused by dementia (see Chapter Two, Q&A#1). Both conditions can co-exist and each merits consideration in its own right.

Assertiveness

After you've acknowledged the hearing loss to yourself and to others, you're then in a position to assert your communication needs in various kinds of situations. *Assertiveness* is a concept that underlies many of the specific steps I'll be suggesting later. You must be willing to inform and educate others about what they have to do in order to make it easier for you to hear and understand. It may be as simple as asking the waiter in a restaurant to turn down the background music, provide you with a written version of the day's selections, or as involved as rearranging the seats at a meeting.

Being more assertive about your listening needs does not come naturally for many people. It may mean changing the habits of a lifetime, but it can be done and it can be quite liberating (there's got to be some advantage to getting older!). Of course, you don't have to take giant steps in the beginning. Even little ones, as long as you take enough of them, will eventually get you to your goal.

Note that you can be assertive about listening needs without being aggressive or hostile. "Would you mind talking a little louder (or a little slower)? That will make it easier for me to understand you," and get better results than, "For Pete's sake, get the mud out of your mouth when you speak to me!" When we assert our hearing needs, we're saying to somebody, "Yes, I really do want to communicate with you," and not simply ignoring them.

Communication Exchange

This brings up the third recurring theme in this chapter: both you and the person with whom you're talking are equally involved in a communication exchange. Presumably, this person wants to be understood as much as you want to understand. Unlike a monologue, a conversation is a two-way street. When you suggest that a seating arrangement be modified, or you inform your conversational partners what verbal modifications to make so that you can better understand them, it's as much for their benefit as it is for yours. What I'm suggesting is that when you work with and help other people communicate more effectively with you, both you and these others benefit. So, acknowledge your hearing loss, be assertive about your hearing needs, and know that you are a crucial half of any communication interchange.

Getting the Most out of Your Hearing Aids

As a hard of hearing person you want to ensure that you're making the best use of your residual hearing. This means maximizing the benefit you're receiving through your hearing aids. Amplification is the only therapy that directly increases the actual amount of acoustic information available. All the training and practice procedures that will be presented are predicated on you first getting as much useful acoustic information as possible through your hearing aids. Although you ought to realize some immediate benefit from your hearing aids, you should obtain even more help after you get used to them. This requires us to consider both some general principles and some specific practice procedures.

Tenacity

Foremost, don't get discouraged! Remember that while you've had a hearing loss for years and experienced the frustrations of poor hearing, for you the sounds you had been receiving seemed perfectly "normal." Now with hearing aids, you're suddenly experiencing sounds that are not only louder, but a different acoustic pattern. You're going to have to reeducate your brain to accept these different sound patterns as the new "normal." As a rather simple analogy, what you now perceive with hearing aids can be likened to someone talking English with a very different accent. Just as it takes time for an American to get used to an Australian speaking English, or for a New Englander to comprehend the speech of someone who comes from the Deep South (and vice versa), so it will take some time for you to adjust to the amplified "accent" coming through your hearing aids. But it can be done.

The Adjustment Process

When you first turn on your hearing aids, you're suddenly going to hear many sounds of which you previously were unaware. Many of these sounds will jog familiar memories. For others, you're going to have to consciously identify the source of the sound, either by asking someone or by honing in on it yourself. One woman in a recent hearing aid orientation group was going a little crazy with the hissing and splattering sounds she kept hearing until she realized it was coming from her frying pan. She hadn't heard the sounds of frying food for many years.

Suddenly you're going to be exposed to a world of sound you had forgotten, such as the whirl of the dishwasher, the whine of an electric can opener, the sounds of birds singing, or the "ting" of your microwave when the food is done. Other familiar sounds will be experienced somewhat differently and may even be disturbing, such as traffic noises in the city, the tumult in your favorite restaurant, and the screeching from your grandchildren's first lessons on a new musical instrument! It's true that it's a noisy world in which we live, and it seems to be getting noisier all the time. But it's the only world we have and it's the one in which you're going to feel more comfortable when you can more fully hear what's going on. But once you know the cause and source of some unpleasant sound, you can then feel free to ignore it or walk away. Knowing what to ignore can be as important to achieve as knowing what to listen for.

Expectations

Not everybody will be able to realize the same degree of benefit from hearing aids. After resisting the notion of hearing aids for years, some people when they finally relent and get them expect that the devices will recreate their hearing abilities of fifty years ago. It doesn't work that way. While hearing aids will help most people with hearing loss, no matter how advanced a hearing aid or how skilled the hearing care practitioner, the ultimate benefits achievable through amplification are determined by the nature of your auditory disorder. I won't dwell on expectations because it's been well covered in previous chapters, but your satisfaction with hearing aids is going to depend greatly on your expectations, which need to be realistic (neither too high nor too low).

Be in Control

A key in your successful use of hearing aids is working closely with the professionals from whom you received the hearing instruments. They can't give you the full benefits of their skills unless you call upon them with your questions, comments and experiences. For new hearing aid wearers in particular, the period right after acquiring the hearing aids is crucial. It is at this time that instances of "Murphy's Law" (whatever can go wrong, will) seem to occur with depressing regularity. Most hearing aid related problems can be solved, or at least minimized, but they won't be if you don't bring them to the attention of your hearing care practitioner. Of all the tales of woe I hear from people regarding their hearing difficulties, unsuccessful attempts to use hearing aids are surely among the most common. It really is a shame; so many people could have been greatly helped and their lives enriched if they had just persisted.

I suggest you wear your hearing aids for as long each day as you feel comfortable, with the eventual goal of wearing them all day every day. But you have to be satisfied that they're helping you hear better and they don't hurt your ears after a few hours. Sometimes, depending upon the nature of what you're hearing, you may want to remove them (e.g., at a hard rock concert or mowing the lawn on a windy day). Go ahead and take them out and don't feel guilty. Remember—you're the boss. You're in control. They're your ears!

Reeducating the Brain

What "getting used to hearing aids" really means is that you'll be undergoing a learning process. Not only will you have to get used to the hearing aids themselves, but you'll also have to get accustomed to a new pattern of sounds. For some people with long-standing hearing loss, the process of reeducating the brain can be enhanced by specific training or fitting techniques. Because you haven't heard certain sounds for a long time, the signals amplified by the hearing aids may sound strident, artificial or just downright unpleasant. It's possible that these unnatural or harsh quality sounds can eventually help you improve your speech perception skills, but only if you can get used to them.

What the hearing aids may be doing is amplifying high frequency speech sounds (like /s/, /sh/ and /f/), elements of which you may not have heard, or have heard differently, for years. Your hearing care practitioner has a good idea of what the final amplification target should be; he or she just can't get there sometimes in one fell swoop. So, don't get discouraged if you're asked to come back for tune-ups. In fact, this may be a mark of an especially conscientious practitioner. Each time you return, your provider may perk up the high frequencies, drop the low frequencies, or do something else to help ease your adjustment to the new auditory experience. While just <u>actively</u> listening to people may be enough to get you used to these new sound sensations, you may also find it helpful to engage in the kinds of listening practice procedures that will be presented later.

Speechreading Principles

Until recently, the preferred term for speechreading was lipreading. We now use *speechreading* to emphasize the fact that when people talk, a great deal of nonverbal but important information is conveyed via facial and hand gestures, body stance, intonation, rhythm of sentences, and the nature of vocal emphasis placed on words and syllables. For example, the phrase, "<u>Where</u> are you going?" conveys quite a different meaning than "Where are <u>you</u> going. And "CONvict" has quite a different meaning than "conVICT," even though the two words look alike on the lips. Lip movements alone are insufficient to clarify the different meanings in these instances. What speechreading is, then, is lipreading "plus." Our goal is not only to understand more of what a person is saying by looking at the lips, but also to be attuned to these other important sources of information. While much of this tuning may be unconscious, it is nevertheless very real. Speechreading will help you whether you have a mild or profound hearing loss.

If you can see a person's lips and you know the language, then you have already been speechreading—to some extent. I'll bet if I asked you if you can speechread, you'd say, "No!" But you do, as the following example will demonstrate.

Ask your significant other to silently mouth a month of the year (one of twelve choices). If you can't get it, try a day of the week (that is, seven rather than twelve choices). If you still don't get it (and assuming your partner's lips can be seen clearly—this is very important to check), ask this person to mouth the lip movements for the numbers "three" or "four." Nobody misses this. So, the chances are that to some extent you've already been speechreading, as long as you can observe the lips of the speaker. But you should do even better if you understand the general principles of speechreading.

Visibility

The first general principle is that you must be able to see the lips of the person talking. Now this not only sounds simplistic, but positively insulting! Of course one has to see the lips in order to speechread. But you'd be surprised how many people with hearing loss who need and can benefit from speechreading do not observe the lips of their conversational partners. They may look them "right in the eye" or simply stare off to one side.

The lip movements we're trying to pick up are minuscule, rapid, and very fleeting. Since our vision is most acute at the point of focus, our best chance of perceiving these cues is by looking right at the lips. Our peripheral vision should be sufficient to detect facial expressions, hand gestures, body stance and so forth because they're larger movements. Try it. Look at someone's lips and note that you can also observe the expression on his or her face as well as any hand movements.

Think about the implications of these simple rules. You will not be able to speechread when:

- in the dark;
- a person's back is turned;
- you're far from a person;
- your visual acuity is poor (so, pay as much attention to your vision as to your hearing);
- a person's mouth is covered;
- your conversational partner wears a full mustache and beard;
- light is in your eyes;
- and the face of the person you're talking to is shadowed.

In other words, any situation that reduces visibility of the lips is going to interfere with speechreading. How often have you or people you know made an extra effort, perhaps unconsciously, to ensure that you can see the person who's talking? If you have, you've been speechreading, even though you may not have known it.

Restricting Lip Movements

Anything that obstructs the movements of the lips is going to hamper speechreading to some extent. Some people seem unable to talk unless they have a pencil or the frame of eyeglasses jutting out of their mouth. Other people talk as if they were practicing to be ventriloquists—their lips hardly move at all! And some people seem to talk with a perpetual smile, making speechreading almost impossible because of the way the smile distorts lip movements. In a few of these instances, a little assertiveness may help, such as, "Please take the pencil out of your mouth" (but not "Wipe that smile off your face!").

But for some people, it's a losing battle. Because of the wide variations in movement of the lips while talking, there'll be large individual variations in the "speechreadability" of people's lips. For people with whom you have a continuing relationship, it's worth reminding them to use more lip movements while talking. Sometimes this works quite well. For the tight-lipped stranger, this may be a futile endeavor. Conversely, you don't want anyone to exaggerate lip movements, thereby adding distortion and defeating your purpose. It may be easier to change the world than the way some people talk. So be realistic. You can't win them all.

Familiarity with the Language

You can't speechread unless you know the language. This also sounds quite simplistic, and in a way it is. If you're trying to speechread someone talking in a language you don't know, of course you won't be able to speechread. But what this brings up is the notion of predictability. Since only about 30-40 percent of the sounds in the English language are clearly visible on the lips, even in the best of circumstances there are lots of gaps that have to be filled in. This isn't quite as imposing a task as it may appear, as long as you and the person you're talking with share a common language. English is very redundant, with many linguistic and situational cues that can help you correctly predict some words you otherwise couldn't. For example, try filling in the blanks in the following sentences:

    A. Please put the dish on the _____.
    B. He hit a home _____ in the last _____.
    C. Where are you _____?
    D. After dark, it snowed again last _____.
    E. I just heard the weather report. They are _____ a major _____ tonight.

In sentence "A," someone could be saying "floor" or "bookcase," rather than "table," but this is unlikely. Sentence "E" is an example of how a previous sentence (or sentences) can improve predictability. The words are "predicting" and "storm." Now—wasn't that easy?

Native language speakers do this kind of thing unconsciously. No matter what language you've grown up with, you can (or could prior to the onset of your hearing loss) effortlessly understand verbal messages. Don't you often fill in the last part of people's conversations before they finish? This is the kind of predictability I mean. If you're not listening to your native language, then you'll have more difficulty making these predictions (as well as more difficulty understanding speech in noise or other difficult listening situations).

Topic Restrictions

The ability to speechread improves when you can reduce conversational possibilities. When you go to the bank, a municipal office, shop in a clothing store or talk to a co-worker regarding a particular project, the topics are likely to be limited by the context. I don't suppose you talk about certificates of deposit in the clothing store, or the weather in Italy at the bank. Basically, "topic restrictions" are another way of employing linguistic predictability.

This is not something you necessarily do consciously. However, the fact that topic restrictions do enter into almost any conversation should make it easier for you to speechread and to keep from making bad guesses. If it makes no sense at all, it probably wasn't the message! Yes, a lot of guessing does take place, and sometimes, as has happened to me, I guess incorrectly (with occasional embarrassment, but just as often a laugh for everybody). Still, I would rather guess and keep the conversation going than give up.

It's the Message Not the Medium

When you're engaged in conversation, don't focus on speechreading particular sounds or words. Instead, attend to the message, i.e., the meaning of what the other person is trying to convey. If you consciously try to analyze the minuscule, rapid and fleeting movements of the lips, you're going to be three sentences behind before you figure out the missing sounds or words—if you ever do. Many books on speechreading spend an inordinate amount of time describing how different sounds of speech are made.

Speechreading successfully, however, does not require you to identify all the sounds a person forms on his or her lips. What being successful means is that you're able to understand what is said.

Because so many of the sounds of speech are either invisible or are formed exactly (or almost exactly) the same way as other sounds (like *maybe* and *baby*), even the most skilled speechreader cannot identify all of them. What they do, and what you must do, is use your knowledge of the language and your awareness of topic restrictions to fill in the gaps. By focusing on the message rather than specific movements, you'll find that subsequent sentences may clarify words that you may have missed.

Hearing

One crucial principle in speechreading is the necessity for you to use your residual hearing as well as you can. Now, this seems like a contradiction! If we're talking about speechreading, why bring up hearing? Well, how often are you talking to someone while you're not wearing your hearing aids? Maybe late at night or early in the morning, but at most other times you're likely to be wearing them. And why would you not wear them if you know they help you? Normally, then, when conversing with other people, you're going to depend on both speechreading and hearing. And that's fine. Because your goal is to understand speech as well as you can, you should use whatever cues are available to help you realize this goal.

As I mentioned earlier, many of the sounds in English are completely invisible on the lips. For example, look in the mirror while saying the word, "key." It can be spoken with no lip movements at all. This is the kind of word that requires context in order to be understood. Now consider hearing the teenager in the house ask: "Why can't I have the _____ to the car!" Even though the word is invisible, there is no misunderstanding what the word was! While you're still in front of the mirror, silently say the words: /pan/, /ban/, and /man/. They all look alike don't they? This is where hearing comes in. It is hearing that allows for such refined differentiation. Fortunately, it's relatively easy to hear the difference between the /p/, /b/, and /m/ sounds, since /b/ is voiced, /p/ is voiceless, and /m/ is a nasal sound (also voiced).

In other words, much of what you can't see, you can often hear. This is an important principle. It turns out that there are many speech sounds that are very difficult to differentiate visually, and yet are relatively easy to distinguish through hearing (i.e., while the /t/, /d/, and /n/ sounds look identical, they can be identified through hearing). Conversely, other sounds that are difficult to hear (like /s/, /f/, /t/ and /th/) are relatively easy to speechread. So, what we find is that vision and audition provide complementary information. What's lacking or difficult to perceive in one sense can often be picked up by the other. It follows, then, that depending only on speechreading or hearing will often limit your ability to communicate. It really does take two to tango!

In real life situations there are always going to be variations in how well you can see and hear someone talking. Noise will tend to mask out many speech sounds and reduce the amount of information you get through hearing. This forces you to depend more on visual cues in order to understand a spoken message. But because the loudness and type of noise constantly vary, these changes will cause your ability to understand speech to vary as well. In some situations you may have to rely almost entirely on vision to understand speech, while in other situations, you may be able to understand even without looking at the speaker. By using both vision and audition as much as possible, and any other sources of information, *most* hard of hearing people can comprehend *most* of what *most* people say in *most* situations. I'm qualifying because there will inevitably be times when you miss part or almost all of a conversation. This will happen. What I'm suggesting is that you think positively. Think of the occasions you can understand rather than focusing on the times you can't.

Practice Procedures

Over the years there have been hundreds of books and articles purporting to teach people how to speechread, often extolling some specific method and providing lots of practice material. Personally, I find the training material more helpful than the theories. Dedicated and persistent practice will help improve just about any skill. I have experienced the benefits of intensive speechreading practice, even <u>after</u> many years of having a hearing loss and using hearing aids. Several years ago, because of an infection in both ear canals, I could not use my hearing aids for about a month and could only depend on speechreading in trying to comprehend speech. Ordinarily, I'm not a very good speechreader; I tend to depend more on audition than vision. But after several weeks of trying to communicate without hearing, mainly with my wife, I found my ability to speechread her noticeably improving. I still couldn't carry on an extended conversation by speechreading alone, but at least in context I was able to carry on abbreviated conversations. (We did cheat once in a while and use finger spelling to clarify difficult words!) So, speechreading practice, with and without sound, wherever and with whomever you do it, can help you improve your understanding of spoken messages.

Tracking

One creative such exercise, termed *tracking procedures*, is practiced in action with a communication partner. Don't be discouraged by the professional jargon. These are basically exercises that require you to comprehend some segment of speech before proceeding to the subsequent segment. In other words, you're required to track through a conversation in a sequential manner. The tracking exercises can be structured so they incorporate other training procedures as well. I'll explain how this works.

You're sitting across from your conversational partner. The room is well lit and you're relaxed. (It's going to be fun!) This person has selected a paragraph as practice material. It can be from the newspaper, from a magazine article, book, or specific material related to one's vocation or interests. Whatever material is selected, it's important that the sentences follow each other in some kind of logical sequence. You should be informed of the general content or topic of the paragraph, as would be the case in real life.

Now, while using a soft voice and normal, not exaggerated lip movements, your partner should read the first sentence of the paragraph to you. Did you get it all? Did you get any of it? Your job is to repeat whatever you understood of the sentence, guessing when you're not sure. You possibly made some errors, but also got some words correct.

If you missed any part of the sentence, the first step is for your partner to repeat the whole sentence again, verbatim. You may or may not get it all this time. If not, what your partner has to do is emphasize the parts/words you missed by making them slightly louder and exaggerating the pronunciation somewhat. When you do get the sentence correctly, your partner then goes on to the next sentence, which is preceded by the sentences already understood correctly. When persistent errors occur, it is time to practice "communication repair" strategies (adding noise via television or radio will enhance the realism of the exercise).

Communication Repair Strategies

In practicing *communication repair strategies* you're focusing on the elements in the communication exchange that have broken down. When you don't understand what's being said, the person you're talking to may not know this, or what he or she can do to correct the situation. But you should, and so you can advise your conversational partner what to do in order to communicate more effectively with you.

The rationale is simple. In conversation, asking "what?" or "huh?" doesn't often help very much. Mostly what people will do when they hear these expressions is to repeat the word of phrase over and over again, maybe just as softly, quickly, or poorly articulated. In other words, they keep repeating the speech pattern you didn't understand in the first place. Your task is to try to figure out why you missed what you did, and then to ask your partner to make specific modifications. Maybe the person talked too slowly, or slurred speech, or talked with his or her hands in front of the mouth, or any number of other possibilities. Perhaps you don't need the entire sentence repeated; maybe all you didn't get was the last word. So you ask the person to repeat only the portion you missed. You might request qualification. "John, you said Sally was out golfing today, but at which golf course?" With a creative collaborator, you can simulate many real-life situations.

Your goal is to practice communication repair strategies enough in a protected situation so that you feel comfortable in utilizing them every day. For example, you can ask a ticket agent at an airport to look at you when speaking, or to talk a little louder, slower, and so forth. When you assist the person you're talking with to be a more effective communicator, you're applying the three themes I spoke about earlier: you're acknowledging your hearing loss, being assertive about your communication needs, and placing equal responsibility for the communication exchange on the person with whom you're talking.

Auditory Training

If we've learned anything in audiology in the past fifty years, it's that the hard of hearing person's perception of speech can be improved with acoustic experiences and auditory training. This has been dramatically illustrated by people with severe to profound hearing loss who have received cochlear implants. Recipients initially often report some strange auditory sensations that they're unable to identify or use. After a while, however, the brain learns to make sense of strange sounds. While new users of hearing aids may not experience anything quite so dramatic, still you're sure to encounter a somewhat altered acoustic universe. It is this modified auditory world that now has to become your new normal.

Adaptations of the previously described tracking procedure can serve as helpful auditory training procedures. In the auditory version, your partner reads the material for you to repeat while his or her lips are covered (no visual cues). For most people, this is still going to be too easy. Since the most difficult situation for understanding the spoken word is in noise, that is how you should structure a listening situation. Use recorded material, such as books on CD, as the noise source.

For example, the first sentence is read. If you miss part or all of it, your partner should, in this order:

- repeat it verbatim;
- repeat it—stressing the words you missed;
- if you still miss it, the sentence should be rephrased, but then go back to the original version for you to repeat;
- and finally, let you see and hear the sentence if you still missed it.

After you get the first sentence, your partner should then read the second one and continue the process throughout the entire paragraph. So I suggest no more than 15-30 minutes in the beginning. As you well know, trying to listen under adverse circumstances can be fatiguing.

Self-Administered Training

Getting and keeping a cooperative partner can be quite a challenge. After a while, you may run out of cooperative partners! Remember though, the purpose of the training procedure is not to endanger relationships, but to foster good listening habits! You can advance toward the same goal working by yourself, using CD recordings of books available at libraries. Listen to the recording initially while following the written version (which requires that the recording be unabridged), and subsequently when you gain more confidence you can listen without the help of the script. Listen to the recording for as long you feel comfortable, but I would suggest no less than 20-30 minute sessions three or four times a week. I also suggest that you use a direct audio connection from the audio player to your hearing aids (or cochlear implant). This can be done with a direct audio connection to the hearing device; earphones placed over ITC hearing aids; or via telephone coils and a neckloop or dual silhouettes. Your audiologist will be able to help you with the set-up.

The purpose of this exercise is twofold: One is to provide you with the experience of listening to the new sounds provided by your hearing aids. It may take time for you to get used to the auditory sensations that you're now hearing, but this listening practice will help you realize the goal. Secondly, this gives you confidence that your hearing abilities can be improved with time and practice. I used this technique extensively myself when I first received a cochlear implant. It was a difficult but challenging task. On the upside, I got to read some books I otherwise wouldn't have!

Computer Controlled Home-Based Audio-Visual Procedures

There are also training procedures for those people who prefer more structured training. This type of program used to be provided by professionals in face-to-face therapy sessions. However, in the past few years, there has been an increasing recognition that the traditional models of auditory and speechreading training are no longer viable, mainly for economic reasons. Face-to-face therapy encounters take time, too much so for traditional third-party payers (Medicare, insurance companies, etc.) to be willing to support. There is clearly a need to develop economically viable methods that are convenient, effective and relatively inexpensive—and can be self-administered at home. Several of these will be reviewed here. There are others, but these are ones I have personally tried and with which I'm most familiar. Each comes with a compact disk and a user booklet. All are user friendly and appear to be based on sound, professional principles (e.g., content, lesson progression, reinforcement). The first is Listening and Communication Enhancement (LACE), an enhanced auditory training program that includes a variety of listening tasks, supplemented by occasional helpful hints regarding effective communication strategies. An explanatory video at the beginning of the program clearly outlines the training procedures. It requires a commitment of some 30 minutes a day, five days a week, for four weeks, although this can be modified somewhat if one wishes. At the conclusion of the program, research studies suggest that speech perception skills can indeed improve. It is recommended that the LACE program be accomplished collaboratively with a referring audiologist who can remotely monitor your progress.

LACE includes five types of listening tasks, each one beginning at a level where success can be assured; then the program proceeds to more and more difficult listening conditions. Each of the five types of stimuli reflects the kinds of situations and hearing difficulties often reported by people with hearing loss. The first such task requires the comprehension of sentences delivered in noise, probably the most frequently reported challenge. Listeners repeat as much of each sentence as they can. The next screen then presents the sentence visually. If the sentence has been understood ("yes" or "no" buttons on the screen), then the next sentence presentation is made more difficult. If it has not been understood, the sentence is repeated. This basic paradigm is followed for all the subsequent listening tasks. (Further information can be obtained at www.neurotone.com.)

The second home-based training program is Seeing and Hearing Speech. As the title indicates, visual cues (speechreading) are added to the listening exercises, thus quite nicely complementing the content of LACE. The program consists of four major groups: (1) vowels, (2) consonants, (3) stress, intonation and length, and (4) everyday communications. Each group is broken down into further subgroups and then subdivided further. For example, the consonant group consists of nine subgroups, each of which contains six additional lessons. All in all, it makes for a great deal of practice material on a single CD. The program permits a user to select either the visual or auditory mode, or both together. A variety of speakers present the stimuli, some easier to speechread than others (reflecting what happens in life).

Users are instantly informed whether they made the right choice. If it's wrong, the user can elect to see or hear the presentation again or just go on to the next stimuli. (Further information can be obtained at www.seeingspeech.com).

The final and most recently developed home-based audio-visual training program is ReadMyQuips. It utilizes a crossword puzzle format and the stimuli are sentences (or quips) spoken by a number of historical figures and contemporary celebrities. Different speakers will say the sentences in varying levels of background noise. Your job is to fill in the crossword puzzle spaces with the words spoken by the speaker. If you get the sentence completely correct, the background noise is increased making the next presentation somewhat more difficult. If the sentence is not completely correct (incorrect words are highlighted), the noise level is reduced making the task easier for the next presentation. It is a challenging and fun task, that helps make an onerous task more pleasant. Further information can be obtained at www.sensesynergy.com.

All training procedures, those with partners and those you practice yourself, are designed to improve your communication skills in real life, outside of the practice environment. As long as you're engaged in effective communication exchanges with people, then you're practicing good carry-over. Remember, your audiologist is a vital resource; do not hesitate to take advantage of his or her professional skills. This is what they're all about (or should be!).

Hearing Tactics

Hearing tactics is a term used to describe environmental manipulations that make it easier for you to understand other people. Using hearing tactics, like military tactics, means you must plan ahead, marshal your resources, and engage the "enemy"—the difficult communication situations. No hearing tactic or hearing device will eliminate all of your hearing problems, but you can take a giant step toward reducing many of them by understanding how you can exert more control over communication. Next are a few examples.

Move Closer

Always try to move closer to the person talking. This is an underestimated but valuable technique. For example, in the average room if you're eight feet from someone speaking and you can move to within four feet of this person, you've increased the sound pressure of the speech signal at the microphone of your hearing aids by about 6 dB. If you can get within two feet of the speaker, then the increase is 12 dB—a rather significant boost. I really don't recommend getting much closer unless you have a special relationship with this individual!

While it's true that some modern hearing aids will compensate for distance by providing more amplification of weaker sounds, and less for stronger sounds, they will also amplify the background noises in a similar fashion. Better comprehension results when the sound you want to hear is located close to the hearing aid microphone, whether this sound is a person talking, a television, radio, or anything else. This will improve the speech to noise ratio (the intensity level of the speech relative to the noise) that is perhaps the most important factor underlying your speech perception.

Quiet the Room

This is a principle that applies just about every place you go. When you walk into a restaurant for a relaxing meal and find that the young staff is playing loud music through the P.A. system, what do you do? Here's where assertiveness pays off. Many young people seem oblivious to loud music in the background—this all seems very normal to them. When it's explained to the staff that the music makes speech comprehension virtually impossible for the person with a hearing loss, more often than not they graciously comply with the request to lower the volume.

When you arrive, look for the quietest table. Seat yourself in the center of your group where it's easy for you to see and hear everyone. Stay away from any extra noise-producing areas such as the kitchen, live or background music, and avoid loud air conditioner or heating system fans. Better yet, look for places to eat that encourage private conversations; restaurants do differ in their sensitivity to noise.

Many people feel that they have to have the stereo turned on when entertaining people in their home. A gentle reminder to turn it down or even off usually suffices. At a family gathering, the youngsters may have the television set turned up while ignoring it; if it's your house, pull the plug and/or move the youngsters to another room. If it's not your house, try diplomacy or try to move your personal conversation to a quieter area in the house. Whatever environment you happen to be in, make sure you have a good sight-line to all the guests. Don't sit at the end of a long couch. You may not see or hear the person at the other end. If only a small group is involved, try to get some conversational rules established. If your social gathering consists of friends, you can ask that only one person talk at a time. Cross-conversation presents one of the most difficult situations for people with hearing loss.

Senior centers and retirement homes, particularly those that serve meals, often present a challenging communication environment. In such places, speech comprehension can be improved by:

- acoustical treatment on ceilings and walls;
- rugs, if possible, on the floor;
- rubber coasters on chair and table legs;
- soft material, such as felt, on dining tables under the tablecloths to reduce the clattering sounds of dishes and silverware;
- or sitting at a smaller (4-person) rather than larger (8-person) table during meals and other activities.

Advance Planning

Plan ahead for any activity. For example, before you attend any large-area listening situation (theater, lecture, house of worship, etc.) call ahead to see if an assistive listening device is available. These devices basically transmit the sound from its source to special receivers (FM radio, infrared, or the telephone coil in your hearing aid). They enhance the acoustical clarity of sounds that emanate from loudspeakers some distance from you. In other words, they serve as "acoustical bridges" from the sound source to your ears.

Most such places are required by the Americans with Disabilities Act (ADA) to have assistive listening devices available. Houses of worship are exempt, but many provide such devices as a courtesy anyway. I personally would not attend any large area listening event without ensuring that such devices were available. Without one, I either don't know what's going on or I'm straining so hard to hear that I don't enjoy the activity or performance.

Microphone Technique

Even if assistive listening devices are available in an auditorium, listening problems can still occur, particularly if the sound source comes from someone using a microphone. What I've observed over the years approaches inconsideration by people who should know better when they use a microphone. What seems to happen is that talkers get so wrapped up in what they're saying, they forget that there's a microphone on the podium. Many microphones require that a talker speak within 6 or 8 inches of it for effective pick-up, otherwise the signal degrades or decays rapidly. Sometimes, if it's a hand held microphone, many speakers wave it around as if it were a baton or a pointer—everywhere but close to their mouth. So what do you do?

- You arrive a little earlier and remind the event organizer, the speaker or the minister, of the necessity for the speaker to stay close to the microphone while talking.
- During the talk, some speakers are going to walk away from the microphone still speaking. You ask loudly (but politely) for the speaker to move closer to the microphone. Other people in the audience will appreciate your assertiveness because of their own hearing difficulty.
- If a lapel instead of a podium microphone is available, ask that it be used and pinned close to the person's mouth.

If there's a public question and answer period after the talk and you can't hear the questions, don't suffer in silence. Ask for the questions to be repeated before answers are given. Remember that you're probably not the only one in the audience who would benefit.

In a recent hearing aid orientation group, I heard of an excellent example of how a bit of assertiveness can help many other people in the audience. One of the participants complained that he never heard the homilies prepared by the same two women in his church. Their voices were soft and they typically sat two feet or so away from the microphone. Every Sunday, he said he just sat there and waited for them to finish, not understanding a word.

His normal hearing wife then piped up and said, "I never understand them either and I don't think anyone else can!" Before the next service, the husband asked the two women to talk right into the microphone since he was having difficulty understanding them. That Sunday, not only my client, but everyone heard the women loud and clear.

Wrap Up

In this church anecdote, we have an example of the three themes with which I began this chapter. The hard of hearing person had to acknowledge the hearing loss, had to be assertive in approaching speakers, and the effort served the purposes of both parties in the communication exchange. The lesson in this example is that you, as a hard of hearing person, must be more than a passive recipient of hearing services. You have to take more control over your own listening needs. Work closely with your hearing healthcare professionals. They have information and skills that will help you.

No—magic wands are not available to wave away your hearing loss, but with the appropriate use of modern technology and the judicious use of appropriate communication strategies, you can go a long way in reducing the impact hearing loss is having in your life.

CHAPTER TEN
Telecoils
And Wireless Assistive Listening
David G. Myers, PhD

Dr. Myers is a Hope College social psychologist (*www.davidmyers.org*) and author of seventeen books, including <u>A Quiet World: Living with Hearing Loss</u> (Yale University Press). Vocationally, he is a communicator of psychological science to college students and the lay public. His scientific writings have appeared in three dozen academic periodicals, including *Science,* the *American Scientist,* the *American Psychologist,* and *Psychological Science.* He has also digested psychological research for the public through articles in four dozen magazines, from *Scientific American* to *Christian Century.* Avocationally, Dr. Myers has authored three dozen articles and an informational website (*www.hearingloop.org*) explaining hearing aid compatible assistive listening.

Imagine a future in which hearing aids had doubled usefulness. While they would serve as sophisticated microphone amplifiers (today's common use), they would also serve as customized in-the-ear speakers for the wireless broadcast of television, PA system, and telephone sound.

Although that second possibility may sound like a futurist's dream, it actually describes the present world in which I live.

My office phone can broadcast "binaural" sound (to both my ears), even if I set it on my desk while taking phone messages.

When I watch the TV nightly news, my TV speakers will broadcast normally for anyone else in the room. Although that sound is too faint and foggy for me to hear clearly, it's not a problem. At the touch of a button, my hearing aids become the TV speakers, broadcasting crystal clear sound customized just for my ears.

When I worship at my church (or at nearly any one of my community's main churches) I need only press that same button and the clergy's voice will be broadcast privately by my hearing aids, which receive wireless sound signals rather like my laptop receiving wi-fi signals.

Although most American readers of this book will have no clue what technology enables this doubled functionality for hearing aids, hearing aid wearers in Britain would immediately know what I'm talking about (as would most such people in Scandinavia, and many in Australia). The simple technology has two parts. The first is the tiny and very inexpensive *telecoil* (or *t-coil*) that now comes with most new U.S. hearing aids. These little coils of copper detect magnetic signals transmitted by telephones.

Telecoils and Telephones

Unbeknown to most people, telephone handsets transmit not only sound, but also a magnetic signal. By federal mandate, all wired, landline telephones manufactured in the United States since 1989 are "hearing aid compatible," as are some cell phones. That means they transmit an interference-free magnetic signal to telecoil-equipped hearing aids. The hearing aid wearer simply activates the telecoil by pushing a button (on a remote device or on the hearing aid). Suddenly, the hearing aid becomes an ear plug, receiving no room sound. Instead it receives and broadcasts a strengthened phone signal. For this reason alone, more and more hearing aids of all sizes and cost levels are now coming with telecoils. Figure 10-1 shows how small telecoils are by comparison to the dime in the picture.

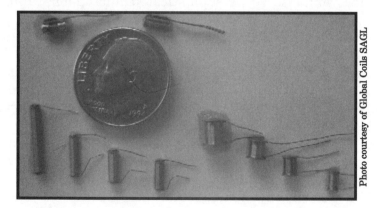

Figure 10-1: assorted telecoils

Hearing Loops

Enhanced phone listening was reason enough back in the late 1990s for my audiologist and hearing aid manufacturer to include telecoils in my hearing aids (for no additional charge). "I would strongly recommend that just about every hearing aid include one," says the influential audiology researcher-writer and American Academy of Audiology Career Award winner, Mark Ross. "It is the position of [the Hearing Loss Association of America] that telecoils be given the prominence they deserve as a valuable hearing aid feature that will allow the expanded use of assistive listening devices," concurs the Hearing Loss Association of America (HLAA). In Britain, where virtually all hearing aids distributed by the National Health Service come with telecoils, the assistive listening use of telecoils is well understood and, as I have witnessed during my annual sojourns there, widely applied.

I first experienced hearing aid compatible assistive listening at the 800-year-old Iona Abbey, off Scotland's west coast. Knowing that I was challenged to understand the spoken sound, and noticing a hearing assistance sign similar to the one in Figure 10-2, my wife nudged me to activate my telecoils. The result was dramatic, the audiological equivalent of going from a rough gravel road to fresh asphalt. Suddenly the speaker's voice seemed to be coming from the center of my head. It was what we psychologists call an unforgettable "flashbulb" experience.

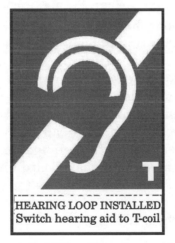

Figure 10-2: symbol for availability of hearing assistance

On one visit to London, I ventured into Westminster Cathedral, where a Saturday afternoon mass was underway. The priest's voice was indecipherable to me after bouncing around the cathedral's vast stone walls. But not a problem, for when I activated my telecoils the priest's voice suddenly was broadcast by loudspeakers that were inside my ears. There was no need for me to locate and wear a conspicuous, hearing aid incompatible headset.

The next morning I worshiped at Westminster Abbey. Once again, the sung and spoken words were a verbal fog, until I switched on my telecoil receivers. With utter convenience and invisibility, the deliciously clear sound transmitted wirelessly via my own hearing aids. When the 50th anniversary of Queen Elizabeth's coronation was celebrated there, the program's first words were: "The whole of the church is served by a hearing loop. Users should turn their hearing aid to the setting marked T."

On an ensuing evening, a taxi drove me to a drop-off point near a theater. As I sat in the back of the taxi, the driver, from the other side of a plastic screen, gave me walking directions. I heard them clearly, because all London taxis (and now many in Edinburgh, I've discovered) have induction loops that broadcast the driver's voice to telecoil-equipped hearing aids. As I paid the driver, I marveled at the technology and asked him where the microphone was. He smiled, and pointed to a little dashboard hole.

After experiencing this new use of hearing aids in many British venues, from churches to the Royal Society of Edinburgh's auditorium and seminar room, I thought why not the USA? To begin bringing the technology home, I did what you can easily do. I obtained and installed a simple home TV room loop. (These can be purchased for $200 or a little more from vendors listed at hearingloop.org/vendors.htm.) One simply (a) plugs the little loop amplifier into a power outlet, (b) connects it using the patch cord provided to the television's audio out port, and (c) runs the loop wire around the seating area. The wire can be run under the carpet, around the edge of the room, at the ceiling or attic level, or, as in my case, by dropping it through the baseboard and then stapling it to the basement ceiling studs. For even greater simplicity of installation, one can purchase a thin pad that slips under the cushion of one's favorite chair, which effectively loops not the room but just the chair.

Once installed, I turned on the TV, activated my telecoils, and found the corners of my mouth approaching my ear lobes. Even with the TV volume set low, sharp, strong sound was broadcasting from inside my ears, at a volume (for me alone) that I set on the loop amplifier. Unlike my previous infrared TV listening headset, which required removing my hearing aids, the new loop system harnessed my hearing aid technology, which includes a mic + telecoil (M/T) setting. Rather than blocking out the sound of the phone or doorbell ringing, or my wife speaking, the M/T setting welcomes such sounds alongside the TV signal. Figure 10-3 shows how this is set up.

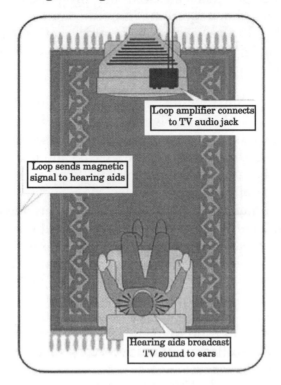

Figure 10-3: magnetic signals surround a room for TV reception

And it's not just me benefiting from this home technology. A California audiologist I know now offers a free home TV room loop with every hearing purchase. (The installations initially were done by his 17-year-old son, using fish tape to snake wire under carpet.) While looping more than 1900 homes, his practice has flourished thanks to word of mouth from his happy patients, who are enjoying doubly useful hearing aids. When he surveyed samples of his patients with and without the home loop system, he found markedly higher satisfaction with both TV listening and with hearing aids among those with the home loop. Given home loops, 63 percent indicated the highest level of satisfaction with TV listening, as did 53 percent regarding their hearing aids. For patients without a home loop system, the corresponding figures were 7 percent and 3 percent.

Looping West Michigan

In the US, the prevalent assistive listening systems are hearing aid *in*compatible. They require us in public venues to locate, check out, wear, and return receivers which often come with conspicuous headsets (which, by the way, loop systems can also provide for those without telecoil-equipped hearing aids).

Your local movie theaters have these. Under the Americans for Disabilities Act, public venues with fixed seating for 50 or more people must provide these receiver/headset units. But rarely if ever do you see them used. People with hearing loss *should* be willing to undergo the hassle and mild embarrassment of using these headsets. But because few of us are willing, and because their generic sound is often unsatisfactory, they mostly sit unused in closets. One manager at my city's seven-screen theater complex estimated that their units are checked out about once a month per theater. The new Nashville Music City Center considered a plea for hearing loops, but decided, "Not enough people asked for individual listening devices at the old convention center to justify the expense of looping the new one." (*The Tennessean*, August 30, 2012).

The Rochester, New York, Hearing Loss Association of America appreciates this reality: "Many people do not extend themselves to identify their need, collect personal receivers ahead of time, or wear rather noticeable headsets. Such receivers are always required for FM and infrared systems." My own church offers a good example of this. Our old infrared assistive listening system was used by one severely hard of hearing person. Within a few months after installing a new hearing loop system, I knew of ten people who were invisibly using it (most of whom approached me to express their delight).

After a community initiative, with support from two local companies and our community foundation (see hearingloop.org), most of my city's major worship and public facilities became looped, including our library auditorium, senior citizen center auditorium, city council chambers, college auditoriums, funeral homes, and so forth. Word of mouth and media publicity has since spread the technology to surrounding cities such as Grand Rapids, where the city convention center, performance hall, and airport concourses, individual gate areas, and outside waiting lounge are now all looped. Signage indicating loop capability at a drive-up bank teller is nicely represented in Figure 10-4. (See hearingloop.org for listings of West Michigan loop installations.)

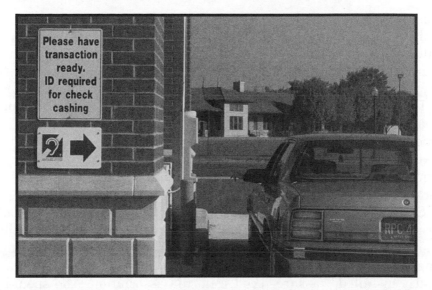

Figure 10-4: driver making bank transaction at drive-up teller window can see signage indicating loop capability and thereby can switch hearing aid from "M" to "T" for clearer reception

Countless unsolicited anecdotes reveal the initiative's human impact. One woman, who refused to use her church's headsets, said, "It's actually fun to go to church, and it hasn't been that way for a long time." After switching on her telecoil and hearing sound "like I hadn't in years," another woman burst into tears of joy. One pastor was initially let down when his church's new loop system had no known users. Within eight months, however, three long absent hard-of-hearing parishioners had returned and three newcomers had sought out his newly accessible church.

The enhanced functionality of hearing aids has motivated many people to visit our area's hearing professionals, who in turn have been supportive of West Michigan becoming a cool place for people with hearing loss. The former owner of Holland, Michigan's largest audiology practice observed that, "Never in my audiology career has something so simple helped so many people at so little cost." Another audiologist I know told me that, "Nearly everyone I've seen who has the loop system has had favorable results."

Looping America

The West Michigan effort is being extended by hearing loss consumer groups in other communities, including Arizona, New

Mexico, Washington, Florida, Colorado, Oregon, Illinois, Georgia, and New York City. In Wisconsin, thanks to the leadership of Dr. Juliette Sterkens, the HLAA's national hearing loop advocate, more than 200 venues in cities statewide have been looped (see LoopWisconsin.com).

In Sarasota, Florida, all seventeen stage theatres are now looped. Hearing Loss Association leader Ed Ogiba (personal communication) reports that "roughly 90% find the loop a superior delivery of sound to any system they previously used. In addition, the loop does not require headsets or a neck loop which many people refuse to wear because of the stigma attached to it."

Speaking for consumers, the Hearing Loss Associations of California and Michigan are now recommending hearing aid compatible assistive listening. "In all new and extensively remodeled buildings, wherever there is a public address system, a loop should be permanently installed," declares the California association. And speaking for hearing professionals, the American Academy of Audiology joined forces with the Hearing Loss Association of America to promote a year-long national "Get in the Hearing Loop" campaign.

Thanks to the leadership of Janice Schacter (who operates New York City's Hearing Access Program) and of Manhattan's Hearing Loss Association, many of the city's major venues now are looped, as are some 450 subway information/token booths. Figure 10-5 is a picture of the New York City Transit Wall Street station, indicating the hearing loop assistance. Under a recent contract awarded to Nissan, all future New York City taxis will come with hearing loops. And more significant installations are in the works (possibly including future U.S. passenger rail and subway cars).

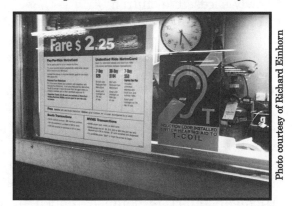

Figure 10-5: NYC Transit Wall Street station loop signage

In the aftermath of recent media attention, including a front page *New York Times* story on the U.S. hearing loop movement, two major A-V suppliers (Listen Technologies and Williams Sound) announced plans to train and equip their hundreds of A-V dealers to do hearing loops. Other loop engineering and installation firms have also sprung up around the US. And Hearing Loop Products has trained nearly 200 people in loop installation workshops conducted across the country.

People with hearing loss, especially those who have experienced the alternatives, prefer hearing aid compatible loop systems because they:

- *do not require picking up*, wearing, and return of external equipment;
- require purchasing and maintaining *fewer receiving units and batteries*;
- are *used invisibly*;
- work in *transient situations* (ticket counters, drive-through stations, etc.);
- entail *no hygienic concerns* regarding multiple users of ear pieces;
- enable *flexible use*, including direct listening (Microphone), loop broadcast (Telecoil), or both (M/T);
- deliver *personalized sound*, customized for one's own hearing loss;
- work with new generation *cochlear implants*, which also are now coming with telecoils;
- are *hearing aid compatible*, and are therefore
- much more *likely to be used*, and increasingly so after installation, which also makes them;
- more *cost-effective* on a per-user basis.

Such considerations led Terry Portis, past executive director of the Hearing Loss Association of America, to conclude that, "Our country will never be accessible for people who are hard of hearing unless we make hearing aid compatible assistive listening a reality." Former Better Hearing Institute director Sergei Kochkin also notes that the way to increase adoption of hearing aids is to increase their utility. You can double their functionality—with simply-operated "miniaturized internal wireless receivers in *every* hearing aid"—and word-of-mouth advertising will promote hearing aids and the stigma of hearing instruments will decline.

New 21st Century Wireless Hearing Solutions

Hearing loops are today's easily affordable wireless hearing solution. Other wireless technologies are now becoming available. One can, for example, purchase wireless FM transmitters which communicate with receivers attached to behind-the-ear aids, though at considerable expense. Might future alternative technologies offer assistive listening that, like telecoils and loops, is *miniaturized* (can work in all aids), run on *low power* (won't require large batteries), *inconspicuous* (unlike the headsets available with hearing aid incompatible assistive listening systems, as well as with loop systems), and virtually *free* (and thus affordable to anyone)?

Why wait to work toward an American future where the functionality of hearing aids is doubled? Wireless assistive listening is available today! Looping America could increase the appeal and use of hearing aids, reduce their unit cost, decrease the stigma associated with hearing loss and hearing aids, and increase public support for Medicaid, Medicare, and insurance reimbursement for hearing aids. If consumers, hearing professionals, audio engineers, and facilities managers can mobilize around this vision, then perhaps the United States needn't forever lag other countries in supporting those of us with hearing loss.

CHAPTER ELEVEN
How to Obtain Professional Help
Robert E. Sandlin, PhD

Dr. Sandlin has served as an Adjunct Professor of Audiology at San Diego State University and as research and clinical audiologist in several clinics and hospitals. He has also served as Director of the California Tinnitus Assessment in San Diego, an organization devoted to developing effective strategies for the non-medical management of those with subjective tinnitus. He has published over 90 articles and edited four major texts on hearing aid sciences and amplification, and contributed a number of chapters to other texts. He has said that his greatest achievement was his many tremendous children and grandchildren who provided a constant source of satisfaction for him and his wife, Joann. Dr. Sandlin unfortunately passed away in 2012. This chapter appears in memoriam and with great fondness.

There are many things you will want to consider in your search for professional guidance. This is especially true in view of the improvements in hearing aid design and function. Advances in hearing aid technology can be very helpful to those with hearing loss.

Why is this so important to you? Hearing aids with computer capability have been available now for several years. They permit the hearing professional to help you in ways that were impossible in those preceding years. The fancy name for this advanced hearing aid technology is *Digital Signal Processing.*

The task of finding the most qualified individual to manage whatever hearing problems you have is not as difficult as it might first seem. Your biggest challenge will be narrowing your search down from a lot of choices to a few options. In doing so, you'll reduce your frustrations and sharpen your focus on what is required. There is always a certain amount of frustration in seeking help for some human ailment. You may have found yourself asking a number of questions in recent years, especially if your hearing has deteriorated. If you've been seeking answers, you've come to the right chapter. Here are some typical questions that new hearing aid candidates ask themselves before they make that first visit to a hearing healthcare practitioner:

- Do I need a hearing aid at all?
- Do I need one or two?
- How do I know if the recommended hearing aids are the best for me?
- How do I know whether the person I'm going to see is competent?
- How do I determine if the person I'm seeing really cares about me or is merely profit-motivated?
- What if I don't like the hearing aids, what are my alternatives?
- How can I determine if medicine or surgery can improve my hearing?
- Do I have to wear them all of my waking hours?

These questions are not uncommon. The important thing is that all of them can be answered in a meaningful way. A lot depends on who you select to be your personal hearing healthcare manager. Your physician can tell if medicine or surgery would help. The audiologist can verify the presence or absence of a significant hearing loss and select and dispense the appropriate hearing aid. Also, the audiologist may provide hearing test results to your doctor suggesting a possible need for medical attention. The hearing instrument specialist is also qualified to select, fit and dispense hearing aids, but is not licensed to conduct a diagnostic audiological evaluation.

Be optimistic about your potential success with hearing aids. Think of all the benefits you could experience. Look at it this way. You've already won more than half the battle just by making a positive decision to do something.

The purpose of this chapter is to suggest ways in which you can connect to the proper hearing care professionals, and understand what they can offer. This will require positive action on your part, defined as taking steps to successfully eliminate or reduce your hearing problem. As usual, the first step is the most difficult.

This chapter will provide guidance to you and your family on several key issues. In the process, it should reduce your fears, apprehensions and frustrations sometimes associated with any search for better ways to manage a health problem. By the end of this chapter, you should be knowledgeable about how to move through the maze of hearing healthcare professionals. You should know who's who in this profession. You should be able to establish who is the best person to meet your particular needs. You'll know how to determine the qualifications of the provider who might best serve you.

If you have doubts or problems regarding the hearing healthcare person you elected to see, get a second opinion. You know your hearing is extremely important to you. You have every right to find the best help possible. Not all hearing health professionals have the same amount of knowledge and experience. Let's review some history underlying the emergence of hearing aid dispensing as an occupation in the United States.

History of Hearing Aid Dispensing

The selection and fitting of hearing aids has been practiced for well over seventy-five years. During that period of time, there have been steady improvements in the design and performance of hearing aid devices. However, less than twenty-five years ago, hearing aid dispensers were not required to have any special technical training to carry out the necessary tasks for selection and fitting of hearing aids. Nor was it required for the individual to have a dedicated place of business, only sufficient capital to buy hearing aids from a manufacturer and go into business were needed. Further, early on, there was no sophisticated diagnostic or hearing aid measuring equipment required to validate the degree of improvement provided by hearing aids or to qualify their acoustic performance.

As the manufacturing of hearing instruments became more technologically advanced, so did the ability to measure their electroacoustic characteristics. As time passed, manufacturers initiated training programs in the proper selection and fitting of their hearing aid products. For the most part, early educational programs provided by the industry were very instrumental in improving selection and fitting skills. The manufacturer was interested, primarily, in its own product and most educational efforts were dictated by that philosophy.

Nevertheless, from the early introduction of hearing aids and the early selection and fitting practices, those who had less than positive experiences regarding hearing aid use developed some negative attitudes. While some of these attitudes may have had a basis in fact, it's important for you to know that significant and positive changes have come about within the hearing aid dispensing field. For example, by the late 1970s, most individuals who dispensed hearing instruments were licensed by the state in which they practiced. In order to receive a hearing aid dispensing license, a test of basic competency had to be passed. It was a rather simple test, but served admirably as a first effort to establish a level of competency.

Today, these tests have become much more sophisticated. Areas of study include a basic understanding of the anatomy, physiology, neurology and pathology of the hearing system. They also include factors contributing to hearing impairment; psychology of the hearing-impaired person; and electroacoustic measurement of hearing aid devices.

In addition, other areas of study include administering and understanding hearing tests; understanding audiometric test results for the purpose of fitting hearing aids; learning effective counseling strategies; and becoming familiar with state laws governing the professional activities of hearing instrument providers. These tests are not exhaustive ones nor necessarily difficult, but did cover basic educational requirements. Licensure to fit hearing aids created a higher level of competence.

There are two individual and distinct disciplines now dispensing hearing aids: the Clinical Audiologist and the Hearing Instrument Specialist (HIS). Let's look at both of these practitioners.

Hearing Instrument Specialists

There are thousands of qualified hearing instrument specialists throughout the United States. State requirements and licensing assures that they are knowledgeable and capable of performing necessary measurements for the selection and fitting of hearing aids. Many are members of the International Hearing Society (IHS). In order to qualify and maintain membership in this group, continuing education is mandatory. The hearing instrument specialist also can pursue additional training to achieve Board Certification (BC) status. In order for members to be board certified, a written examination must be taken and passed. This examination is more demanding of specific knowledge than is the examination of individual states. In order to obtain maximum objectivity, the Board Examination is managed by a group not officially affiliated with the International Hearing Society.

It can be stated positively that the hearing instrument specialist is much more qualified to select and fit these devices than they were at any time in the past. This qualification has been largely based on state licensure and mandatory continuing education requirements. Much of the credit is due to the continuing efforts of the International Hearing Society and its board certification program. Additionally, state certification has advanced the professional status of the hearing aid specialist and has inspired greater consumer confidence.

History of Audiology

Although the medical profession has long been interested in the measurement of hearing loss for the purpose of diagnosis and treatment, there was no great effort until World War II to establish a separate branch of medicine dealing solely with the objective assessment of the human auditory system. At that time, hundreds, if not thousands of returning servicemen had incurred permanent Physicians recognized the value of assessing hearing because of its implications regarding medical management. It soon became evident that most hearing loss caused by battle conditions could not be treated medically or surgically. This was so because most of the injuries to the ear were caused by shell blasts and other loud, explosive noises. As an aside, do you know that once hearing nerve cells are dead, they cannot be regenerated? I mention this because the majority of people with hearing impairment have received damage to the ear, which causes some of the nerve cells to die.

Because of the number of servicemen and women with hearing loss, there needed to be some organized clinical program. A program was needed which could evaluate the type and degree of hearing loss as well as develop effective rehabilitation programs. Just the sheer numbers of servicemen needing immediate attention gave need to program development. Advanced techniques of measuring hearing loss were introduced. More sophisticated equipment was developed for the measurement of hearing. Much attention was given to rehabilitation programs that would permit, as much as possible, the hard of hearing serviceman to live effectively in a hearing world. You can imagine the important role that hearing aids played in the successful rehabilitation of these servicemen and women.

Coupled with the urgency to meet the needs of the hard of hearing soldier was the need to provide expanded training for personnel working in rehabilitation programs for hearing-impaired veterans.

As training programs were established and proved to be very worthwhile, a name—a professional label—had to be associated with those who performed these services. A branch of special education merged with medicine and this new academic discipline emerged as the profession of Audiology.

Since those beginnings in the early forties, the practice of audiology has expanded tremendously. The amount of audiological research is reflected in the number of scientific journals devoted solely to its study. The growth of this field is evident by the significant increase in academic programs in hearing science.

It's noteworthy that audiologists have been responsible for almost all of the formal research efforts involving hearing aid use and function. Yet, they were prevented from dispensing hearing aids for profit by their national association, the American Speech-Language-Hearing Association (ASHA).

But all businesses, whether medical or not, are profit driven, and rightfully so or they could no longer afford to keep their doors open. In the early 1970s, many audiologists recognized this. Whether it was naive of ASHA or an outdated ideology, the time had come for hearing aids to be part of clinical audiology practice. Several clinical audiologists in the United States opposed the majority viewpoint and began to dispense hearing aids. They believed they had the right to include dispensing in their responsibilities to consumers. Those audiologists who dispensed hearing aids had their clinical certification revoked by ASHA.

However, by 1978, as more and more audiologists had adopted the dispensing philosophy, ASHA revised their Code of Ethics and accepted hearing aids as being an integral part of the services offered by audiologists. Since that time, audiology has had an enormous and positive influence on the hearing aid industry. Hearing aid evaluation and subsequent dispensing of hearing aids are now considered to be well within the scope of practice for audiologists. The audiologists were well-trained academically, but lagged behind in management skills and the 'selling' of hearing instruments. This deficit no longer exists.

Clinical Audiologists

Audiologists are familiar with the functions of the human auditory system and trained to understand normal and abnormal functions of that system. They are trained to perform routine and at times highly technical diagnostic tests to determine what is causing abnormal auditory function. Their depth of understanding of the physiology, neurology, anatomy and pathology of the auditory system is greater than that of the hearing instrument specialist. This is true because of the required education.

Furthermore, audiologists provide rehabilitation to those with hearing loss ranging in degrees from mild to profound. Over the past many years, the field of audiology has expanded to include the assessment of hearing loss for the purpose of selecting and fitting hearing aid devices.

The advanced training and educational requirements are dictated by ASHA. To previously obtain a Master's Degree in Audiology, typically six years of study at an approved college or university were required. In addition, the student must have served a clinical fellowship year and passed a rigorous examination. Audiologists had to earn at least a Master's Degree to assume clinical or academic responsibilities. Master's degree are no longer granted. However, several universities have offered a Doctor of Philosophy (Ph.D.) degree as the terminal degree requiring two to four years of additional study. For those audiologists wishing to pursue teaching and research, the Ph.D. in audiology still remains a good direction in order to learn those skills.

In the mid-1990s, there was a concerted effort by a group of audiologists to establish one common professional degree by which all "clinical" audiologists would be recognized—the Doctor of Audiology (Au.D.). Today, the most common degree granted by most audiology programs is the Au.D. Academic preparation stresses the diagnostic procedures required to differentiate various pathologies of the auditory system. This may include anything from wax in the ear canal to a tumor resting on the eighth cranial nerve. For most academic programs, audiology also includes rehabilitation programs for the deaf and hard of hearing.

Also, academic programs relating to the electroacoustic performance, selection, assessment and fitting of hearing aids have been added to the curriculum. Inclusion of hearing aid dispensing as an integral part of audiology practice began in the early 1980s and has continued to grow in acceptance. One cannot stress too strongly the positive implications of the AuD. The curriculum is designed to emphasize the diagnostic and clinical skills needed to manage a private practice—not unlike the medical professional—and to enhance clinical skills, including hearing aid dispensing. Therefore, the Ph.D. in audiology is for intentions of research. The Au.D. is intended for clinical purposes.

Similarities among Providers

In those states requiring licensure, both the audiologist and hearing instrument specialist must pass the same mandatory examination and complete the required number of continuing education hours each year to maintain licensure. Members of both groups must abide by the same standards of ethical practice and are subject to the same state laws governing the dispensing of hearing aids. (Did you know that in states where licensing is mandatory, the physician must also be licensed to dispense hearing aids?)

One significant similarity is that each group has access to the same hearing instrument manufacturers and to all literature and clinical information pertaining to hearing aids and their electroacoustic performance. There are no restrictions placed on which manufacturer can provide hearing aid devices to those who dispense. There are, however, a few manufacturers of hearing instruments who will sell their product only to approved franchises. The basic philosophy underlying a given franchise operation is that it's more efficient for the manufacturer to deal with persons dispensing only their product.

Obviously, there are pros and cons to this argument, but very active franchises do exist in today's marketplace. All practitioners have access to pertinent scientific and trade journals and may very well modify that which they do in the selection and fitting process based on information contained in specific articles. Most hearing instrument dispensers and dispensing audiologists have more than a single brand of hearing aids available to their clients.

From a humanistic point of view I think you'll find each discipline is sensitive to your needs. Most individuals will do his or her best to satisfy your needs and maintain your confidence in their abilities.

A Difference among Providers

The major difference as already alluded to is that of formal education. The hearing instrument specialist does not have a formal educational background in measuring the performance of the human auditory system for purposes of diagnosis or in the rehabilitation of those with hearing impairment. He or she is more typically required to have a high school education in order to sit for the examination to qualify as a hearing instrument specialist. This description of their academic requirements is not intended as an indictment of the qualifications necessary to become a provider, nor is it intended as a yardstick against which to measure proficiency in the selection and fitting of hearing aid devices. Rather, it's a straightforward statement of criteria imposed by states in granting licensure to those qualifying by examination to dispense hearing aids. There are thousands of qualified hearing instrument specialists throughout the United States. By far, the majority is knowledgeable and capable of performing necessary measurements to select the most appropriate hearing instruments.

The education required to become a clinical audiologist is extensive. It entails undergraduate and graduate school training in assessing neurophysiologic function and dysfunction of the hearing system through the administration of defined clinical tests. Audiology is, and has been for decades, a recognized academic discipline. Inherent in the training of audiologists is courses relating to hearing aid amplification. A number of training institutions provide clinical practicum for their graduate students in hearing instrument dispensing and specific courses relating to selection and fitting of amplification devices.

Your Significant Other

When starting your search for qualified service providers, it may be wise to consider taking another person with you. It can be your spouse or another family member or friend. This person can be a second pair of eyes and ears to assist in the evaluation process. He or she may be able to provide a somewhat more objective observation of the hearing care provider's skills and services. This person can serve as a sounding board to respond to such questions as, "What do you think I should do?" or "Should I get one or two hearing aids?"

Finding the Preferred Professional

In the selection of a qualified provider, you want someone who demonstrates proficiency and competence. You must realize that you'll be using hearing aid amplification for many years to come, and therefore, will want to establish a long-term relationship with whomever you choose. This is something to which you should give considerable thought.

Listed below are some of the recommended criteria you can use to select the best person in whom you can place confidence and trust. These are the essential features you should look for when seeking a hearing care professional.

Expectations of Your Hearing Care Provider

Hearing aid researchers agree that the interaction of the hearing aid fitter and the client is a critical element in successful hearing aid use. There are specific elements to this important relationship that are common to providers who achieve a high degree of satisfaction among their clients. Successful providers believe in the benefit of hearing aids and they keep up with rapid changes in hearing aid technology.

Expect your hearing health provider to have an attractive and clean office with convenient business hours. Expect him or her to act professionally, and to be knowledgeable and demonstrate the benefits presented in the next section. You should have hearing aid options explained to you in simple terms. Demonstrations are often helpful that allow you to listen to a particular type of circuitry, to compare different settings in noise, or to experience the difference between monaural (one hearing aid) and binaural amplification. A good professional dispensing hearing aids never assumes that clients cannot understand complex concepts. You should be given as much information as you require in the form of discussion, CDs or DVDs, books, brochures, consumer guides and technical articles. There's a popular phrase that suggests "too much information" may not be good. There's a time to stop giving information. Not all patients want or need a bus load of materials. Information needs to be tailored to your needs.

Research has identified that stigma is still a common reason why some people resist purchasing hearing aids. It's very important that you're allowed to express your feelings about how hearing aids will look and what you think about them. Simply talking about your feelings associated with your hearing loss can be of tremendous benefit. Some people don't care what size or style of hearing aid is chosen. Others are overly conscious about the cosmetic aspect. However, hearing aids today can be manufactured so tiny as to be essentially inconspicuous and even entirely concealed.

Experienced providers know how to motivate skeptical, timid hearing aid candidates. They know that proactive clients have a higher likelihood of becoming satisfied hearing aid wearers. All providers want their clients to be willing to go the distance, even if they make a few mistakes in the beginning. Sometimes the process can be difficult. A caring professional will always see you through, if you will.

Optimizing the match between your lifestyle and communication needs is an important determination by your provider, something which can have direct impact on you. We're all more likely to trust someone who we feel understands us. Therefore, effective hearing care providers are good listeners. It's important that your provider takes the time to learn what problems you have in meetings, groups, theater, with co-workers, family, and in your place of worship. It's also important for you to express what you hope to improve in your hearing world as a result of amplification.

Once you've been fit with hearing aids, it's absolutely mandatory that the person who fit you with the hearing aids explains in detail how to care for hearing aids, how to clean and maintain them, how to use the switches or remote (if there is one), and how to change batteries. You should receive an instructional booklet for later referral after the initial counseling or instructional session.

Especially with programmable hearing aids, it's not uncommon to come back several times in order to get "just the right fit" (physical, acoustical, audiological) for you. This is a normal part of the hearing aid fitting process. Multiple adjustments to hearing aids are normal and are not indicative of a "lemon." However, it's important that these adjustments occur during the trial period, and that you're satisfied the product meets your needs.

Years of Service

If somebody has been providing hearing services for many years, it generally is an indicator that many people with hearing loss have been seen by that person. Although it may not necessarily indicate superior knowledge and care, it does suggest that this person has been in business awhile and is not likely to disappear tomorrow. As with any skill-related work, the longer you do it, the more proficient you become.

In the selection process, you may want to determine the years of service a particular practitioner has in providing amplification devices to those with hearing loss. However, I must tell you that years of service does not always mean that the person is the most qualified to work with, or the one who understands the latest in technological advances in hearing aid performance. Don't hesitate to ask anyone from whom you are seeking advice and direction to review his or her professional and academic background.

Level of Knowledge

It's in your best interest to determine the level of skill one has in the selection and fitting of hearing aids. Just having a state license to dispense hearing instruments does not guarantee that the individual is current with technological advances in hearing aid performance. As with many technologies, improvements happen with time. You should not feel uncomfortable, and the provider should not feel challenged, if you inquire about his or her level of knowledge as it pertains to current hearing aid selection and use.

As a matter of fact, many hearing instrument providers may display a variety of certificates indicating they've taken specific courses of study to become more competent. You should take advantage of this by noting the dates on these certificates. A certificate hanging on the wall may not tell you how much the person learned, but it does indicate that he or she continues to study. If you observe there is nothing to indicate continuing education, simply ask what his or her continuing education has been because state licensure now requires it in every state.

Empathy and Compassion

Your hearing aid needs are best met by an empathetic person who understands what you're experiencing. There's really no substitute for empathy. If the hearing health professional is truly empathetic to your needs, you will achieve the greatest benefit.

Although similar in meaning, compassion is a deep sympathetic concern or feeling for a given condition or for an individual, while empathy is more of an intellectual acceptance and understanding of an individual's need or given condition. In essence, you want services rendered by someone who really understands how you feel.

Temperament and Likeability

For our purposes, temperament can be defined as the natural and predictable behavior of an individual. As it relates to one's needs when searching for answers to hearing problems, it is the overt actions of the individual. By this I mean that the hearing health professional should display patience, understanding and concern, without eliciting fear or unrealistic statements regarding hearing aid use.

Certainly, knowledge of hearing aid dispensing is fundamental to doing business and meeting hearing aid needs. But a very important and essential ingredient is also the temperament and likeability of the one with whom you are doing business. Likeability is a sense of joy or contentment in the presence of an individual who expresses a sincere interest in your needs and feelings. It is not something that can always be expressed in concrete terms. It's something you feel and experience in a very positive way.

The sense of feeling positive about the hearing healthcare professional cannot be regulated by a state agency. Like a physician with good bedside manners, you want a professional with conduct that allows you to feel protected. You want this person to be sensitive to your needs. You want to feel comfortable revealing your very private feelings regarding hearing aid use. You don't want to feel like you're intruding, but rather, that the hearing health professional appreciates the opportunity to serve you. It's in your best interest to gather a good sense about the person with whom you're expected to work closely.

Dependability

Although seldom discussed in hearing aid literature, dependability is a very important attribute to successful patient management. That is, as a patient, can you depend on your hearing healthcare professional to be there when you need him or her? Does their office have scheduled hours? Is the dispenser there every day of the week or just on certain days? Does the dispenser provide emergency care just in case something goes wrong with the hearing aid? You may consider talking to others who have purchased hearing aids from the dispenser and question them about dependability of the provider.

The large majority of dispensers are dependable. They're interested in providing services when you need them and want you to feel free to call them when a need arises. To the dispenser, it's simply good business practice to maintain a high level of dependability.

Talk to Successful Users

It was stated earlier in this chapter that all hearing losses are not the same. Regardless of the degree and type of hearing loss you may have, others with permanent hearing loss can tell you of their experiences with a given practitioner and whether or not they were satisfied with the services offered and the benefits received. Ask people who have utilized hearing aids for several years. They have experienced the contributions and limitations of technological advances in hearing aid design and performance. They can be a rich resource for you. Be careful though, because the positive experience of one person does not mean you will have a positive experience with the same hearing aid or the same professional. Conversely, the negative report by a friend doesn't preclude you will also have a bad experience. The emotional and physical needs for all with hearing loss are not the same. You may differ a great deal in your emotional reactions, as well as your acceptance and use of hearing aids.

Make it a point to talk to your friends and others who use hearing aids. Not only can these folks be supportive of your pursuit and use of amplification, but you may learn from their positive, real life experiences how best to adjust to and benefit from hearing aid amplification. You may also learn a great deal from their mistakes.

Background Check

As would be true in any profession, if you're uncertain about the audiologist, hearing instrument specialist or the physician providing services to you, contact the Better Business Bureau in your community or directly contact the state committee responsible for hearing aid licensure. You may also check with the IHS, ASHA or AAA (listed in Appendix II.) Normally, these types of complaints have to do with ethical concerns regarding certain questionable actions of the professional.

Further, in many states, hearing instrument specialists and audiologists have their own Ethics Committee. By contacting this committee, you can find out if complaints have been registered against a given provider and how such complaints were resolved.

Spur of the Moment Decisions

At times, some people proceed with a hearing aid evaluation and the subsequent purchase of hearing aids on a spur of the moment decision. Such a spontaneous reaction in some people is exactly what is required to get the task done. But much will depend on your own temperament. If you're a person who doesn't like to spend a lot of time mulling things over and you know what you need, such an impulsive decision to take quick action may work well for you.

On the other hand, someone else may need more time to think about a plan of action. Some people may have to muster the courage (or even the finances) to do something about their problem. That's okay. A few extra days of deciding what course to follow or how to arrange it won't make any difference. No doubt it has taken you years to get to this point anyway. You'll find the professional person who will meet all qualifications you need and demand.

Background Checks

Some consumers consult the yellow pages, go online or select the individual whose advertisement is most visually attractive or largest, or the individual who seems to have the best credentials. Others may select the first business beginning with "A." The value of your background check is for you to ascertain "who's who" in your community. Examine your options and proceed with optimism and faith in yourself that you have discerned the best choice.

Medical Practitioners

Many people prefer to begin their hearing healthcare journey with the family physician who they've known for years and whose judgment they trust. This seems like an intelligent decision because you would believe that your family physician would refer you to a hearing aid provider if needed.

However, as Dr. Carmen previously pointed out, many physicians do not refer their patients to hearing healthcare practitioners for the purpose of obtaining hearing aids. Most of these well-meaning physicians *falsely* believe you cannot be helped. If this has been your experience, I suggest you seek a second opinion (from an audiologist or hearing instrument specialist). Most general practice physicians are not current with state-of-the-art hearing aid technology, and fail to recognize the benefit they provide to hard of hearing people.

Nevertheless, if something about your ears or hearing is in need of specific medical attention, you could be referred to a medical specialist whose primary concern is the diagnosis and treatment of impaired hearing and diseases of the ear. Such a specialist is an otologist. The otologist restricts his or her practice to problems associated with the auditory system. The otolaryngologist is also a specialist in treating diseases of the ear, but treats nose and throat disorders as well. While either can provide you with adequate treatment, otologists are even more specialized in their training.

If your physician or medical specialist refers you to someone for hearing aids, it should be safely assumed that the practitioner knows you will receive competent care. If you have any doubts about such a referral, you should ask your referring source whatever questions are on your mind.

Medical Necessity

There are certain conditions that require you being seen by a medical specialist. By applying these guidelines, you'll have a more informed idea of when a medical specialty evaluation is necessary. According to the Food and Drug Administration, your hearing care professional must consider these criteria before fitting you with hearing aids and take appropriate action if needed:

a) A visible congenital or traumatic deformity of the ear. Many of these are accompanied by hearing loss, and most can be improved both functionally and in appearance.

b) A history of active drainage from the ear, particularly if it's foul smelling. Except for earwax, most drainage from an ear is caused by active infection. Left untreated, the infection can cause permanent damage.

c) A history of sudden or rapidly progressive hearing loss. Except when caused by a plug of earwax, a sudden loss of hearing needs careful evaluation, especially if it occurs in one ear.

d) Acute chronic dizziness, particularly "spinning," is caused by a problem in the inner ear, and may be associated with a hearing loss.

e) Unilateral hearing loss of sudden or recent onset within the past ninety days. The sooner one seeks treatment, the more hopeful the outcome.

f) A conductive hearing loss (air-bone gap on audiometric testing) of at least 15 dB at 500, 1000 and 2000 Hz. Such a hearing loss can usually be restored with medical treatment.

g) Visible evidence of a plug of earwax or foreign body in the ear canal. Such an obstruction is best removed using careful extraction rather than irrigation.

h) Pain or discomfort in an ear. This is usually caused by infection in the external or middle ear. Medical evaluation and treatment usually result in rapid resolution of the pain.

The Medical Waiver

If you're an experienced hearing aid wearer and you're being issued new hearing aids, federal law does not mandate that a physician see you. This is because the government takes for granted that by now you're experienced enough to recognize the presence of a problem, which needs medical attention. New users may not be as knowledgeable. In light of potential problems, federal law requires that anyone dispensing hearing aids be able to recognize a number of fairly obvious conditions of the ears. If a medical condition is recognized by your provider, you can be assured that you'll be referred for treatment prior to issuance of hearing aids.

If you're a first-time hearing aid wearer, federal law allows you to visit a hearing aid provider without first being seen by a physician, so long as you sign a waiver of medical evaluation for hearing. This essentially states, "You are being advised that the Food and Drug Administration has determined that your best health interests would be served if you had a medical evaluation by a licensed physician prior to purchasing hearing aids."

The waiver serves two solid purposes. First, it alerts you, the consumer, to the fact that a potentially serious medical problem could exist and should not be overlooked, especially if you have any ear symptoms. Second, if you were recently seen in a physician's office and you know there's nothing wrong with your ears (other than hearing loss), you shouldn't have to go back through the medical route to obtain approval for a hearing aid. Many consumers feel that a medical visit under these circumstances is both unnecessary, even redundant, and simply adds to the cost. By signing the waiver, you exercise the right to make your own decision.

A Hearing Evaluation

There are a number of hearing tests that an audiologist or hearing instrument specialist can do to determine how severe you're hearing loss is. Please keep in mind that all tests administered are necessary in order to make the most appropriate assessment of your hearing and find the best approach to meeting your hearing aid needs. In essentially all cases, you should have no pain or discomfort during the administration of diagnostic tests.

Please note that all tests performed are for the purpose of selecting and fitting hearing aids. The primary purpose of a hearing aid evaluation is simply that of determining whether you're a reasonable candidate for hearing aid use. Another purpose is that of determining the type of hearing aid most appropriate to your needs.

Otoscopic Examination

Prior to the administration of hearing tests, your hearing healthcare provider should perform a routine otoscopic examination. Its purpose is to visually examine the status of your ear. It takes only a few minutes to complete and can add an understanding to what may have caused your hearing loss. The otoscope is a hand-held instrument about the size of a standard flashlight. It casts a sharply focused light into the ear that illuminates the canal and reveals its condition. Some are connected to a large-screen monitor enabling you to also see.

Some otoscopes have greater magnification and provide the examiner with a more precise view of anatomical structures. Such views may suggest problems that need to be attended to. For example, a build-up of earwax may be viewed blocking sound from entering the ear. Naturally, the greater the skill and training of the professional performing the otoscopy, the greater the chances are that existing problems will be identified.

Another major contribution of an otoscopic examination is that of assessing the status of the eardrum. For example, there could be a hole in the eardrum due to some traumatic incident or disease process. The size and location of the perforation can affect one's ability to hear well enough to understand all that is being said. Furthermore, otoscopic examination can detect the presence of fluid in the middle ear space. Middle ear fluids can greatly reduce your ability to hear sounds at a normal level. Unfortunately, middle ear fluids can become diseased through bacterial invasion and cause serious medical problems.

Please keep in mind that an otoscopic inspection by an audiologist or hearing instrument specialist is not a diagnostic procedure. Only a qualified physician can do that. But if the hearing health professional sees something suggesting a medical condition, he or she must refer you to a physician.

Listening for Tones

Following otoscopic examination, a number of specialized hearing tests may be conducted. The purpose of hearing tests is to determine how much hearing loss you have, if any, and what the probable cause is. Usually, the basic hearing test consists of sitting in a sound-treated chamber, listening to a series of tones and indicating to the professional when you've heard them. Some tones will be low frequency (low pitch) and others will be high (high pitch). As you know by now, if you have a hearing loss, you won't be able to hear all of the tones at normal intensity levels. Also, you will not know how well or poorly you've done until the test is completed.

The lowest tones that the human ear can detect are very close to the sensation of feeling. At the other end of the continuum, a young healthy person can hear tones even higher than the highest violin note. We don't actually need to hear at either of these two extremes, but we do need hearing intact in the middle range where speech sounds vibrate.

Most people have greater difficulty hearing high frequencies. This is readily demonstrated by listening to (without looking at) someone repeat vowel sounds that are all low frequency, such as /a/, /e/, /i/, /o/ and /u/. Now have them produce the utterance of higher frequency sounds that make up consonants like /sh/, /ch/ and /s/ for example. Sixty-five percent of audible speech intelligibility comes from consonant (high frequency) sounds. Putting all of this in context, have someone repeat the words /sheath/, /cheap/ and /sheet/. If you can't hear the very subtle differences between these words, you'll readily appreciate and recognize how important every sound is in adding information to what you hear. You might now also suspect a high frequency loss.

Listening for Speech

As you well know, there's a direct correlation between the level of your hearing loss and your ability to understand words when presented at normal speech levels. Therefore, a couple of tests will be performed to assess your ability to understand selected words. The Speech Reception Threshold (SRT) test entails repeating two-syllable words such as "hotdog," "baseball" or "downtown."

On this particular test, the more familiar you are with the words, the more accurate the results (you just won't be able to predict which order the words will come). These words are presented at progressively weaker volume levels until you're forced to guess at what you think the words are. The value of this test is to determine how soft certain words can be made before you can only repeat them correctly 50 percent of the time. This point is called threshold. It's used as a working reference for the amount of power that eventually will be needed in your hearing aids, and can allow a certain degree of predictable success you may have in their use.

Another test is the Word Discrimination Score. Fifty one-syllable words such as "wet," "chew" or "car" are presented for you to repeat. The lower your score, the greater your difficulty in hearing and understanding people who talk with you. Usually a score poorer than 88 percent would indicate that you have at least some difficulty in some situations. None of the words on this test will be repeated if you miss them. The number of words repeated correctly reflects how well you understand speech under ideal listening conditions. Word discrimination tests are basic to good clinical practice. These tests tell us what your ability is to understand speech without hearing aids.

Assessment of Middle Ear Structures

In a complete diagnostic evaluation of your hearing, other tests may be carried out to determine how well your hearing system is performing. Typically, clinical audiologists conduct these tests on highly sophisticated equipment. In certain cases, it may be important for your practitioner to know if the eardrum is moving appropriately when sounds strike it. If some disease or pathology affects the way in which the eardrum (or other structures) moves, then we want to be able to identify and measure it.

Special diagnostic equipment is used through which primarily two objectives are accomplished: mobility of the eardrum (assessed by increasing air pressure into the outer ear canal), and integrity of the inner ear (by means of a series of loud tones to try to trigger your acoustic reflex). Both the pressure tests and presence or absence of the acoustic reflex add information to the final diagnosis of your hearing problem.

If these basic hearing tests confirm a loss of hearing or abnormal function, then further testing, including x-rays, blood samples, or certain brain function tests may be conducted to gain even more specific information about your hearing difficulties and what may be done about them. The purpose of these various tests is to compare your results with standardized norms. By making this comparison, your practitioner can quickly determine if you have normal hearing or some degree of loss.

Since you might have already suspected hearing difficulties anyway, these tests will confirm your suspicions. Even though some people are apprehensive in general about taking tests, let me assure you that these diagnostic procedures recommended by your audiologist or otologist can be critical in arriving at a competent diagnosis of your problem and its proper management. In most cases, sophisticated tests are not needed to determine your hearing status or the type of hearing aids best suited to meet your needs. So, don't be overwhelmed by all these tests. They're a necessary part of your quest for better hearing.

Medical and/or Surgical Treatment

In many cases, hearing tests, along with other significant information that the audiologist has done, may indicate the need for medical or surgical management. For the most part, this is good news, for it means that such intervention could resolve your problem and restore your hearing to a normal or near-normal state. If such is the case, there is usually no need for hearing aids. However, let's assume you've seen the otologist and are told that nothing medically or surgically can be done to treat your hearing loss. What can you now do to improve your ability to hear and understand? In the final analysis, when a hearing loss exists that cannot be successfully treated by medicine or surgery, the use of hearing aid amplification is the recommended path to follow.

In some cases, there may be a serious condition of the ear(s) that demands surgical or medical intervention before considering hearing aid use. If you think you're having a serious problem or if your hearing care practitioner recommends that you see a physician, definitely do so.

Conclusions

I have discussed many things you may experience in your search for professional care. It can be a highly rewarding journey if you initiate the process for help. The first step in receiving help is looking for it. And little help can be offered if you fail to deal honestly with the problem. Be assured that you'll be rewarded in your willingness to use amplification by significantly improving your ability to understand much more of your acoustic world. Your frequent requests to have conversations repeated should be markedly fewer, and your blueprint to secure a bridge to healing can at last be fulfilled.

CHAPTER TWELVE
Tinnitus: A Journey of Discovery
Grant D. Searchfield, PhD

Dr. Searchfield received his PhD in Audiology from The University of Auckland where he is currently Head of Audiology and Director of the university's Hearing and Tinnitus Clinic. He has published research papers in diverse areas of tinnitus study including auditory physiology and sound therapy. Dr. Searchfield is a regular contributor to international conferences on tinnitus management, and is a member of the Scientific Committee of the Tinnitus Research Initiative.

Tinnitus (ear noise) is a common complaint poorly understood by most people and often misrepresented as a minor nuisance. It's true that for many people tinnitus is a very occasional slight irritation, but some people do suffer and are tormented by the sounds within. While there's still no cure for tinnitus, now more than ever there's a wide range of options for its management and treatment. Since the Third Edition of this book, development of miniaturized computer technology and new understanding of tinnitus has resulted in some tinnitus treatment innovations. In this chapter, I'm going to take you on a journey of discovery, from tinnitus onset through to recovery. The information presented here should help you, your family and friends understand tinnitus and options for treatment. On this journey, I'll introduce some of the most recent treatment ideas and things you can do yourself to reduce tinnitus annoyance. In reading this I hope you'll discover what tinnitus is, how it is managed and signs that you're on the right track for tinnitus recovery. Along the way I'll offer some useful tips to help you on your journey.

Tinnitus is hearing a sound that isn't present in our environment. The phrase "ringing in the ears" is sometimes used, but a ringing sound is just one example of different perceptions that can be classified as tinnitus (buzzing, hissing, cricket sounds are heard alongside many other sounds). A lot of people experience some degree of tinnitus. The American Tinnitus Association (www.ata.org) estimates that as many as 12 million Americans are sufficiently affected by tinnitus that they should seek professional help. Although some people see tinnitus as a by-product of our noisy, stressful modern life, tinnitus has accompanied ear injuries throughout human history. Theories have abounded as to its origins. It was once even attributed to supernatural or religious causes.[1] With development of science and modern medicine, tinnitus became linked to hearing loss. It's now considered not to arise just as a sound signal at the ear, but instead is considered to be the end consequence of a cascade of events, usually commencing with acoustic injury. Tinnitus is the result of a complex interplay of different regions of the brain.

How Tinnitus Develops

Most people with tinnitus have a hearing loss. This sometimes can be quite minor, and the tinnitus sound is often associated with areas responsible for hearing of similar normal sounds. While hearing damage is a common element in most cases of tinnitus, it's only part of a complex puzzle. Increasing evidence from studies of how the brain works suggests that processing within the auditory pathways enhances changes in output from the *cochlea*—the complex portion of the inner ear necessary for hearing. Activity of the hearing system is altered enough to create an image of sound that's actually not there. This is why tinnitus is sometimes called a phantom sound. Scientists believe that some tinnitus is created by a disruption in the balance of inhibitory (stops or slows) activity and excitatory (increases) activity. These inhibitory and excitatory processes emphasize irregularities in auditory activity. The persistent altered input to the central auditory system is believed to eventually result in functional changes in the *auditory cortex* (hearing center of the brain), perhaps so that it becomes synchronized to the new activity. Simply stated, it appears that the central auditory pathways overcompensate for ear injuries (even very small ones) creating tinnitus.[2] In other words, tinnitus is a reflection of a change in the auditory system. After hearing damage, the brain attempts to adapt to the new pattern of acoustic input. Over time, the hearing pathways change their function. This can be rapid or slow. The capability of the brain to change over time is known as plasticity.

The impact of tinnitus on how well we feel is not fully explained by the amount of hearing injury. There's usually a weak relationship between the extent of hearing loss and tinnitus impact. More hearing loss does not mean worse tinnitus. The brain's system responsible for emotion, called the limbic system, is strongly implicated in tinnitus perception and understanding this has become an important part of many treatments.[3] It's thought that much of the severity of tinnitus relates to your psychological response to the abnormal perception. Things that we often don't consider part of the hearing process, such as stress, anxiety and depression, can all lead to more severe tinnitus. Traumatic life events (e.g., death of spouse, loss of employment, ill health) frequently coincide with reported awareness of tinnitus.

Because neck and head movement can alter tinnitus, it's believed that an important contributor to the sensation of tinnitus are brain centers that receive both hearing and somatosensory (touch) activity. Tinnitus can be considered to be the result of many interlinked parts of the brain "network" that includes hearing, other senses, attention, memory and emotion. If just one part of the network is activated, a person might just hear tinnitus. If all parts are activated it may become extremely annoying and upsetting. When we hear tinnitus, what we experience is determined in part by what the tinnitus sounds like, what sounds are present in the background, our attention and distraction, and importantly by who we are as individuals. Since tinnitus is so complex, treatment needs to be approached from many perspectives.

First Steps

When tinnitus first begins, it's common for people to search for the source of the sound. "Where is that buzzing coming from?" I had one tinnitus client who was convinced that crickets were all around his house. Only when he was in boat fishing in the ocean did he realize that the sound was coming from his ears! It's difficult to understand and to accept head sounds. This difficulty in coming to terms with tinnitus is, at least in part, due to it being unlike any other sound in our environment. Normally, once we've localized a sound and determined it is not useful to listen to, we ignore it. But tinnitus does not have an external source that can easily be disregarded. Instead, almost automatically, we keep listening to the sound trying to attribute a cause or source. Feldmann[4] wrote about this in a very philosophical consideration of how we hear tinnitus. He described five categories of reality: The first category of reality included objects that can be perceived by more than one sense (e.g., objects that can be seen and heard). The second category of reality included objects that can be perceived by one sense (e.g., sound). The third category was objects that cannot be perceived directly by the senses without technology (e.g., television). A fourth category was those objects not in the environment, but real, (such as memory of objects). A final fifth category of reality included objects that can only be heard by the individual (e.g., tinnitus). It was suggested that the more real an object (category 1 and 2), the more natural and acceptable it is. Feldmann felt if the source of tinnitus could be identified and made into a form that a person could appreciate in the same way we appreciate normal sound, tinnitus might cease to be a problem.

It is natural for us to be concerned about this strange tinnitus sound. If you've never experienced it before, it can be scary: What's causing it? Is it going to get worse? Am I losing my hearing? Am I losing my MIND!? While there's good information on the Internet or in books (such as this one), the journey to tinnitus discovery should begin with a visit to your family physician. Why? Since tinnitus is unusual, some people have difficulty moving it from the forefront of attention to being a background sound. A consultation with a physician may identify causes of tinnitus that can be treated and most importantly rule out causes that have other effects if left untreated. When you visit a physician or other health professional, take a list of questions with you, and don't be afraid to ask them. Positive information that's based on good evidence may lead to many worries being laid to rest. If we worry about tinnitus we'll naturally pay it more attention. In cases of unexplained tinnitus or tinnitus that's affecting how you feel, your family physician may refer you to an *otologist* (ear surgeon), *audiologist* (science dealing with hearing) or *psychologist* (science dealing with the mind and emotional processes).

The Physical Exam

Physicians will initially ask many questions about your health; when tinnitus began and whether it was associated with illness, hearing loss, injury, medication, balance problems and stress. Blood tests and imaging (brain scans) of the ear and hearing pathways may be used in an attempt to discover a possible cause. In the vast majority of cases the underlying cause has no long-term effects on health. So what are some causes?

Occasionally a physician can hear tinnitus. This is called *objective tinnitus* (somatosound), and is rare. In this case, a physician will try to determine if the sound heard comes from disrupted blood flow, high blood pressure, the neck or jaw, or the *Eustachian tubes* (auditory tube connecting the throat to middle ear) amongst many origins.

It is more common that the tinnitus cannot be heard by anyone other than the individuals themselves. This is called *subjective* or *true* tinnitus. This type of tinnitus is usually, but not always, associated with some degree of measured hearing loss. Middle ear problems such as glue ear and otosclerosis (an inherited progressive hearing loss that results from new bony growth in the middle ear) can result in a stiffening of middle ear bones. Conductive hearing loss may also result from something as simple as earwax blocking the ear canal. Middle ear disease can result in tinnitus because the hearing loss can block exterior sounds from stimulating the ear normally.

Inner ear injuries (sensorineural hearing loss) usually result in damage or dysfunction to the cochlea's sensory structure, reducing hearing nerve activity. This is most often identified as the cause of tinnitus. The most common reasons for sensorineural hearing loss and tinnitus are noise-exposure and aging. Another cause of tinnitus from inner ear damage is from medications toxic to the ear (ototoxic drugs). Your physician will be able to inform you if any medication might contribute significantly to your tinnitus. *Ménière's disease* is another possible cause of tinnitus. It is characterized by episodes of roaring tinnitus, vertigo (spinning dizziness), fluctuating hearing and feeling of blocked ears (see Chapter Three, Q&A#9). Another common cause of tinnitus is injury to the head or neck. Even relatively minor head injuries and whiplash can result in tinnitus. In some people, tinnitus can be turned on and off by exaggerated jaw movement, pressure to the head, and eye movement. Temporo-mandibular joint (TMJ/jaw joint) disorder is also associated with tinnitus. Many people with tinnitus can affect their tinnitus by strong tensing of muscles in the head or neck region. Tinnitus can arise from many other conditions which is why a thorough evaluation by a physician is so important.

One note regarding seeking help from general practice physicians rather than audiologists or otologists—by far most GPs are not trained in this specialty, and although well-meaning, may tell you to just "learn to live with it." While this is good advice, the best advice comes from <u>knowing how</u>!

Treatment Options

Tinnitus is best managed by a "multi-disciplinary" team (many different types of practitioners), so several treatment options can be provided to suit you. In small towns you may not have access to every option, but most practitioners are able to refer you to different treatment providers. The practitioner you see should consider how each aspect of tinnitus affects you in order to select an appropriate treatment plan. You can help the practitioner by considering what aspect of tinnitus is causing problems, what the problems are, identifying the issues and ranking them from biggest problem to least; this can help identify the focus of initial management. This process can help you and your practitioner identify treatment goals and how to work toward them.

Medication or Surgery?

When medications are prescribed for tinnitus, the intent is usually not to treat the sound, but instead to reduce or limit the associated psychological effects such as depression. Sometimes antidepressants are recommended as a first step in gaining some control over the effects of tinnitus, but some types of medication can be counterproductive because they're addictive and may reduce the effectiveness of some other treatments we discuss below. Your physician should be able to give you good advice on what medications, if any, might be beneficial. They will want to treat or manage high blood pressure, thyroid problems, and diabetes. Some doctors may recommend that central nervous system stimulants such as caffeine (in coffee, chocolates and cola drinks) should be limited, however evidence from a study published in 2010[5] suggests stopping caffeine consumption does not improve tinnitus. A change in diet may result in some reduction in tinnitus for some people, but not everyone. If you have a poor diet and/or a link has been found between tinnitus aggravation and a particular food or drink, it's probably wise to make a change. Many "natural" remedies and herbs are advertised to help tinnitus, but there is no good evidence they help. If you're thinking of trying any natural medicine, check with your physician that they won't have negative impacts on any other medications or health issues you may have. In my office, patients have brought me bottles of bizarre folk remedies. While I understand people's desire to search for a silver bullet to cure the problem, I suggest you're best served by having faith in your practitioner. If, as we hope, medications for tinnitus do become available, you can be fairly confident that practitioners will be the ones first aware of them.

New surgical approaches designed to electrically stimulate nerve pathways to modify tinnitus-related activity have been developed and are undergoing trials for use in humans, but surgery carries risks and so may only be appropriate for extreme cases of tinnitus that can't be helped in other ways.

A Comprehensive Audiology-Based Approach to Tinnitus

Audiologists are often the lead provider of tinnitus treatment. The treatment plan will normally consist of assessment followed by counseling and some form of sound therapy. This process will be described in the next sections.

Assessment

Most audiologists will undertake a thorough evaluation of hearing with all new tinnitus clients. In addition to normal hearing tests, a tinnitus evaluation can be useful. Audiologists will differ in the tests they prefer, but typically they'll test hearing levels at very high frequencies, so as to identify any hearing injury missed in standard tests. They'll measure pitch, loudness and the ability to cover (mask) tinnitus. Tests of tinnitus are not particularly precise nor do they really help identify its cause, but they do allow the practitioner to understand what you experience and to consider the types of sound that might interfere with your tinnitus. These tests can also help provide some context for the tinnitus; that is, making it more real for you. A test for *residual inhibition* might be considered (temporary cessation of tinnitus following masking). In this test a loud (usually hissing) sound is introduced to the ear(s) for a minute or so. When the sound is turned off the tinnitus may be reduced for a period. The presence or absence of this reduction does not indicate whether any given treatment will succeed, but when it does reduce the tinnitus, it can be very encouraging to have a period of reduced (or no) tinnitus and indicates the powerful effect that sound alone can have. This will be further discussed later. Tests for loudness discomfort may be used to determine if there's any unusual intolerance to sound. *Recruitment* frequently accompanies hearing loss. This is a phenomenon whereby a slight increase in the intensity of sound results in a disproportionate increase in the sensation of loudness.

Counseling

Once a physician has treated any underlying disease or illness, emphasis shifts to treatment of the tinnitus. Many audiologists offer counseling as a preliminary management strategy. Normally, time is spent to help the patient come to terms with their tinnitus. Knowledge is a powerful ally while uncertainty can lead to anxiety. It is not helpful to think about tinnitus as a worst-case scenario. The information received in a counseling session can be a contributing factor to whether tinnitus becomes a minor annoyance or a significant distraction. If the mechanisms of tinnitus are understood and fears are addressed, less attention is required by the tinnitus. If insufficient information is provided, the void can be filled with fear and concern leading to dwelling on the negative impact of tinnitus and its possible causes. This added attention will raise your awareness of the tinnitus, and its negative effect on your quality of life will be accentuated.

Referral to psychology may be necessary before or alongside other tinnitus management. Seeing a psychologist is important when sufferers react very poorly to their tinnitus, becoming depressed or experiencing anxiety. The counseling that an audiologist provides should not be confused with that provided by qualified psychologists. *Cognitive Behavioral Therapy* (CBT) is a successful tinnitus treatment practiced by psychologists. This approach differs from the information-based counseling undertaken by the family physician, otologist or audiologist—it teaches self-control techniques that can be used to manage tinnitus. Cognitive behavioral therapy involves modifying beliefs and emotional reaction to tinnitus. Sometimes the way we think about things can be very counterproductive, serving only to exaggerate the effect of tinnitus on daily activities. Strategies on how to stop focusing on tinnitus are provided in CBT. Psychologists may incorporate other techniques to assist their therapy including relaxation techniques, stress management and *biofeedback* (e.g., teaches relaxation by monitoring muscle tension). If you're reluctant to see a psychologist, self-help books, online resources about relaxation and relaxation training recordings can be utilized, but they don't provide the support that a good psychologist can. In any case you're encouraged to learn relaxation exercises and to try not to focus on the unpleasant aspects of tinnitus.

Tinnitus can aggravate sleeping difficulties. I know when I don't get enough sleep I get grumpy, and am more likely to worry about work and feel generally glum. Poor sleep commonly accompanies tinnitus. If this happens to you, try to develop a healthy bedtime routine, leave your worries in another room, make sure you go to bed tired, make the bedroom a comfortable place to sleep, and don't drink coffee or cola for several hours prior to going to bed. If you can't sleep, get up and do something. Don't lie in bed and dwell on the tinnitus. If the sleep environment is too quiet, tinnitus may be all that's audible and there's generally little else to take attention away from it. You should be encouraged to play sound in the background continuously through the night to reduce tinnitus audibility. Many people benefit from use of a tabletop sound machine or music player in combination with a pillow speaker for this purpose (described later).

Self-help tips:

- Surround yourself with enjoyable sounds.
- Learn what your tinnitus sounds like—then listen to the world around you.
- Don't focus on your tinnitus—do something fun instead.
- Set yourself some goals that don't involve tinnitus.
- Develop a bedtime routine that helps you relax before going to bed.
- Learn some relaxation techniques such as deep breathing and muscle tensing and relaxing.

Sound Therapy

Sound therapy is the use of sound to reduce tinnitus or its effects in a positive way; the sounds are "therapeutic" in some way. As a general rule, a person with tinnitus should avoid silence (even if that's what is craved). The quieter the environment the more likely the tinnitus will be heard. We can turn this around and say that having sound around you is likely to make tinnitus less audible. Hearing aids do this by turning up sounds that are already there and perhaps even enjoyable. A different approach is to introduce new sounds. As our knowledge of factors involved in generating and maintaining tinnitus have developed many new sound therapy approaches have come about. While many of these new ideas have yet to be proven effective, they do hold promise. Before considering different types of technology that can be used for sound therapy, let's consider some of the ways sound therapy might work. Attention away from tinnitus, intended or not, is likely to be a factor influencing sound therapy success in all cases.

Masking

Masking is the sound therapy method in which tinnitus is covered (or camouflaged) with an external sound to interfere with its clarity. Totally covering the tinnitus is not always possible but partially masking the tinnitus can often occur. Masking may allow you, the sufferer, to determine when you don't wish to hear tinnitus. Benefit comes when the masking noise is more pleasant to listen to than tinnitus. For example, a hissing masking sound may resemble rain, and some people find imagining a rain shower more relaxing than just listening to tinnitus. Practitioners differ in their approach regarding setting the level of the masker relative to the tinnitus. Some advise complete masking of the tinnitus. Other practitioners try to partially cover it. Masking occurs because the brain has difficulty separating signals containing similar information. In some cases tinnitus may be quieter or disappear for a period of time following a masker being turned off. This reduction is called residual inhibition, or post-masking relief, mentioned earlier. If residual inhibition occurs it can last for as little as a few seconds to several days. Residual inhibition is interesting from a research perspective because if we could learn how it occurs (we don't know for sure yet) we might be able to use sound in new ways to extend its effect or even make it permanent.

Habituation Therapies

Another way to use sound is to train the brain to disregard tinnitus. If the tinnitus is made less obvious, habituation (or sustained filtering) of the tinnitus may occur. *Auditory habituation* is a reduction in perception of familiar and uninteresting sound. In our daily activities habituation is the process that allows us to respond appropriately to stimuli that are important (like hearing our name in a crowd) while ignoring sounds that are unimportant (like the humming sound of a refrigerator or computer). When a sound fades into the background of consciousness, it has become habituated. The goal of habituation therapy is to relegate tinnitus to being an uninteresting background sound. Initially, benefit from sound therapy devices occurs only when they are worn; the sound reduces contrast between tinnitus-related sounds and normal auditory activity. In 6-18 months if a program of continuous use is followed, the tinnitus may no longer be a problem.[3] Long-term interference of tinnitus perception using sound therapy may force the tinnitus into being a low level of activity relative to the new background sound. This decreased contrast could lead to permanent changes in the auditory processing of tinnitus, leading possibly to its elimination.

Gain and adaptation

Gain is a term that refers to an increase in signal, like a volume control. *Adaptation* is a term that is used in different ways by biologists, neuroscientists and psychologists; here I use it to mean change due to experience. Hearing loss leads to a decrease in auditory information heading to the brain. The brain seems to try and compensate for this, but a negative consequence is increased in noise—heard as tinnitus. *Gain adaptation* is a potential mechanism underlying sound therapy in which the sound reduces the brains volume control for tinnitus.[6] Interestingly perceptual adaptation is dependent on factors such as memory and personality that have been also been implicated in tinnitus.[7]

Neuromodulation

Sometimes neuromodualtion is the word used to explain how treatments affect tinnitus. *Neuromodulation* essentially means brain (neuro) variation (modulation). With respect to tinnitus treatment, it refers to something that is changing brain activity. Most sound therapies must change brain activity in some way, but here we use it to mean a long-term change in neural activity, such as the organization of the brain, particularly its firing patterns that code sound. One outcome of stimulation of the auditory system with tones or in a frequency-specific manner may be some form of reorganization.

Sound for Relaxation

Tinnitus can be a contributing cause or consequence of stress, anxiety and depression. Relaxation can have a positive effect on how we feel. Counseling and psychology can teach us how to relax; some sound therapies also target relaxation. Music and some computer-generated sounds have relaxing qualities. These sounds may activate regions of the tinnitus brain network associated with emotion.

Sound Therapy Devices

Masking and habituation therapies can be implemented using any device that makes sound: hearing aids; ear-level sound generators; combination instruments (hearing aids plus sound generator); tabletop maskers; radios; compact discs (CDs); MP3/iPod devices; and musical instruments. Some other therapies, particularly those attempting neuromodulation, may require a specific pattern of sounds and require a specialized device. Each sound therapy may work in a number of different ways (as described previously); it is difficult to say which mechanism is responsible for beneficial changes seen. In the section that follows I concentrate on the most common devices used for tinnitus therapy. I have deliberately not named specific products or brands. A good practitioner should guide you to the most appropriate therapy available for your particular tinnitus and circumstances.

Hearing Aids and Cochlear Implants

In the presence of hearing loss, the fitting of hearing aids enable auditory input to return to more normal levels. Hearing aids are one of the most established devices for treating tinnitus, their value being recognized since the 1940s. Today's hearing aids can be very effective in reducing tinnitus when programmed and used properly.[8] For the most part hearing aids have been thought to help tinnitus by reducing the stress associated by straining to hear, by diverting attention away from tinnitus to other sounds and by partially masking or suppressing tinnitus with amplified background sounds. The sounds amplified by hearing aids may directly interfere with the hearing system's processing of tinnitus. The frequency-specific amplification provided by hearing aids should interact with the auditory system's excitatory and inhibitory effects leading to the gain adaptation and neuromodulation (described earlier). Think of hearing aids as a form of "physiotherapy for the ears" and use sound to exercise the auditory parts of the brain. The use of hearing aids as a successful sound treatment for tinnitus is dependent on them being physically comfortable, avoiding loudness discomfort and allowing maximum amplification of soft sounds while adequately amplifying loud sounds.

The ability of modern hearing aid technology to compensate for hearing loss across many environments should reduce the stress associated with straining to hear and focus attention away from tinnitus. Successful hearing aid fitting for tinnitus begins with the selection of the correct hearing aid features.[8] When selecting hearing aids for tinnitus management, I like those that give me flexibility to change as many features as possible. In particular I'm looking for hearing aids that allow quiet background sounds to be amplified, not reduced. Quiet sounds are helpful while loud sounds may make tinnitus worse. Injuries to hearing that lead to hearing loss and tinnitus most often first affect the outer sensory hair cells of the inner ear. These cells normally act to amplify soft sounds. When the outer hair cells are damaged it is the soft sounds that first go unheard. If hearing aids can be set to mimic normal function of the ear, quiet sounds can be made to keep the hearing system busy.

In many hearing aids there are features designed to reduce background noise, which is great if you want to focus on speech sounds, but these features are best turned off for sound therapy. Another feature that has only recently become available in hearing aids is Bluetooth. This is a short-range wireless communication system used by computers, mobile phones and in consumer electronics. This allows devices to talk to each other without wires. Many high-end digital hearing aids now offer the ability to wirelessly connect to compatible digital music equipment (e.g., iPods and MP3) and mobile phones. Sounds can be sent from the player to a transmitter that then sends the signals to the hearing aids.

If tinnitus appears to come from one ear, but both have hearing loss, we still recommend two aids. A hearing aid in each ear helps to normalize input to the hearing system that may be better at interfering with the image of tinnitus in the brain. Sometimes I see people who are reluctant to try hearing aids because when they've tried them in the past and experienced discomfort to sound, that seemed to make their tinnitus worse. Often I've found that those hearing aids have been set to overly amplify sounds. The most appropriate hearing aid is one that stimulates the hearing system with quiet environmental sounds, improves hearing for speech and avoids discomfort to sound. Your audiologist should choose features that are desirable for tinnitus management—namely those that enhance perception of quiet environmental sounds without sacrificing comfort.

My research group and associates have undertaken a number of different studies investigating the effectiveness of hearing aids for tinnitus. On average those people who had hearing aids fitted showed close to 40 percent reduction in tinnitus. It appears the people most likely to succeed using hearing aids for tinnitus reduction have good hearing for low-pitched sounds and low-medium pitched tinnitus. Combination aids (described later), might suit persons with poorer hearing and/or higher pitched tinnitus.

Sometimes tinnitus accompanies a total loss of hearing in just one ear (known as a dead ear). Using sound in a dead ear to mask tinnitus does not work, since the masking sound cannot activate the hearing pathways. But sometimes tinnitus localized to a dead ear can be partially masked or reduced by sound in the opposite ear. A sound generator can be fitted to the hearing ear or a special type of hearing aid can be used that transmits sound from the non-hearing ear to the hearing ear. When hearing aids become ineffective due to the extent of hearing loss, cochlear implants become an option (see Chapter Three, Q&A#10). The brain then needs to learn how these signals relate to speech and other important sounds. The upstream effect of cochlear implants on tinnitus is probably a similar mechanism to hearing aids, masking, habituation and neuromodulation. Your audiologist or physician should be able to advise you whether a cochlear implant is a viable option, but with present technology, you would need to have at least a severe hearing loss to generally qualify.

Sound Generators

Sound generator is the term now often applied to the device once called a "masker" or "white noise" generator. They're hearing aid-like ear-level devices that typically produce a hissing sound. Sound generators are often used for persons with tinnitus and normal or near-normal hearing, while combination devices are used when tinnitus accompanies hearing loss. Sound generators are used for masking and long-term use may lead to habituation or gain-adaptation mechanisms of tinnitus reduction.

Combination Hearing Aid and Sound Generator Instruments

If you have moderate hearing loss or want greater control over how much tinnitus you can hear, combination instruments may be more suitable than hearing aids alone. For moderate hearing loss the hearing aid may not be able to amplify soft sounds enough to interact with your tinnitus. Masking sound from a built-in sound generator combined with the hearing aid can be used to reduce tinnitus. Some practitioners recommend combination aids whenever tinnitus accompanies hearing loss. In the Third Edition of this book I predicted that we would see some interesting developments in this technology. Most major manufacturers of hearing aids now have some form of combination devices. These new devices combine the latest in hearing aid design with sounds other than just white noise. Some devices use a series of chimes that have a music-like feature which may have some masking effect, but also are intended to promote relaxation. Other devices increase the level of therapeutic sounds automatically when in a quiet environment and modulate the level of sound in an attempt to draw attention away from the tinnitus. We don't know which strategy works best yet, but it's likely to depend on what suits individuals rather than being a blanket rule. An advantage of combination hearing aids and sound generators over some of the other tinnitus treatment devices is that the single device helps both hearing and tinnitus.

Music Therapy Devices

There are some experimental methods and commercially available devices that use music as the therapeutic sound. Because of its strong emotional associations, music may have more of an effect on reactions than noise-like sounds. Sometimes music is used initially with other sounds to mask the tinnitus, and then weeks later, music alone is used. The idea is that when the level of therapeutic sound is reduced, tinnitus will be heard, but in the presence of pleasant sounds, so that the sufferer can adapt to the tinnitus without being threatened by it. Because tinnitus is so often associated with hearing loss, one manufacturer of tinnitus devices has a product designed whereby music is adjusted so all its parts are audible.

Tabletop Devices and Personal Music Players

Simple tabletop sound machines can be obtained through electronics retailers, local tinnitus support groups and audiologists. These devices typically allow the listener to choose from a range of pleasant environmental sounds (e.g., surf, rain, waterfalls). Personal music players can also be utilized. At nighttime these devices can be used with pillow speakers—small speakers designed to be placed under your pillow or incorporated into their own pillow. Music is an excellent self-help sound therapy option. Listening to classical music is one of the easiest and most common sound therapies. Only music that induces positive feelings should be used. Sad or depressive music may only reinforce a bad mood. I recommend music be played at a low level, ideally where it begins to blend with the tinnitus. These self-help sound therapies don't take into account the presence of hearing loss and are not tailored to an individual's tinnitus. While they are not accompanied by the counseling a practitioner can offer, they can be effective.

Neuromodulation Specific Devices

Some new therapies specifically try and change brain-related tinnitus activity. These therapies typically use tones of different pitches or vary the timing between sounds in an attempt to reorganize representation of tinnitus activity or to change the synchronization of nerve firings representing patterns of tinnitus activity. As our knowledge of tinnitus expands I expect we will see more of these therapies designed for specific types of tinnitus. Such therapies are not yet widely available.

Journey's End and Future Treatments

Everyone's tinnitus journey is different and so is the end destination, but the destination should be one where tinnitus is no longer having the negative impact it had before taking the steps discussed in this chapter. The key to defeating tinnitus is understanding. Sound therapy is part of the practitioner's toolbox, but it can't be used in isolation. Counseling is essential and it is also important that you take some responsibility by applying self-help strategies. Your practitioner should be able to provide you with a clear explanation of your tinnitus and how any therapy works, don't be afraid to ask questions and want more information. My experience is that most people will know within a month if the treatment they're trying is going to be of benefit, but long-term benefits may take much more time.

You may ask when is the tinnitus journey over?

- When it becomes something you don't think about every day.
- When you suddenly realize that you haven't heard it for a while.
- When you no longer listen for it.
- When you can go to bed without it.
- When it's just not a problem anymore.

Table 12-I below presents an overview of the variety of tinnitus sound therapies and potential underlying mechanisms of effect. There is some overlap in how different devices affect tinnitus. Multiple mechanisms may be occurring at the same time.

Device	Possible mechanisms	Help hearing?
Hearing aid	Masking, habituation, listening effort, gain adaptation, neuromodulation, attention	Yes
Sound generator	Masking, habituation, gain adaptation, relaxation, attention	No
Combination instrument	Masking, habituation, listening effort, neuromodulation, relaxation, attention	Yes
Music based	Masking, habituation, neuromodulation, relaxation, attention	No
Table-top/music player	Masking, habituation, relaxation, attention	No
Neuromodulation	Neuromodulation, attention	No

Predicting the future of tinnitus treatment is difficult. When people ask me about the future, I always say there are already effective tinnitus treatment strategies and they should not wait for a cure. Although progress seems slow at times, scientists are making advances. Drugs and neurostimulation methods using electrical or magnetic stimulation of the tinnitus network are under development, but have yet to be proven truly effective on their own. Tinnitus is so complex that there is not likely to be a single cure; rather, treatments may have to be tailored to suit the individual, and may be a combination of medications and sound therapy. Remember for most people tinnitus does not affect their lives. By understanding what tinnitus is, managing any hearing loss and applying the strategies described in this chapter, tinnitus should be reduced to a minor annoyance.

Patient Resources

- American Tinnitus Association
  www.ata.org
- Australian Tinnitus Association (NSW) Ltd
  www.tinnitus.asn.au
- British Tinnitus Association
  www.tinnitus.org.uk
- Hearing and Tinnitus Clinic of the University of Auckland
  www.clinics.auckland.ac.nz

- Tinnitus Association of Canada
  www.kadis.com/ta/tinnitus.htm
- Tinnitus Research Initiative
  www.tinnitusresearch.org

References

1. Stephens SDG. (1984). The treatment of tinnitus—a historical perspective. *Journal of Laryngology and Otology* 98: 963-972.

2. Eggermont JJ & Roberts L. (2004). The neuroscience of tinnitus. *Trends in Neurosciences* 27(11): 676-682.

3. Jastreboff PJ & Hazell JWP. (1993). A neurophysiological approach to tinnitus management. *British Journal of Audiology* 27: 7-17.

4. Feldmann H. (1991). Tinnitus—reality or phantom? *Tinnitus* 91, Aran J-M & Dauman R. Proceedings of the Fourth International Tinnitus Seminar, Bordeaux, France, Aug 27-30. Amsterdam: Kugler Publications: 7-14.

5. St. Claire L. et al. (2010). Caffeine abstinence: an ineffective and potentially distressing tinnitus therapy. *International Journal of Audiology* 49: 24-29.

6. Noreña AJ. (2011). An integrative model of tinnitus based on a central gain controlling neural sensitivity. *Neurosci & Biobehav Rev* 35:1089-1109.

7. Searchfield GD, Kobayashi K & Sanders M. (2012). An adaptation level theory of tinnitus audibility. *Front Syst Neurosci* 6 (46), 10.3389/fnsys.2012.00046.

8. Searchfield GD. (2006). Hearing aids and tinnitus. In RS Tyler (Ed.), *Tinnitus Treatment: Clinical Protocols* (p. 5). New York: Thieme.

Further Reading

Vernon J. (1998). *Tinnitus: Treatment and Relief.* Needham Heights, MA: Allyn & Bacon.

Tyler RS. (2008). *The Consumer Handbook on Tinnitus.* Sedona, AZ: Auricle Ink Publishers.

Acknowledgements

The Tinnitus Research Initiative and the JM Cathie Trust have supported this author's tinnitus research. He has undertaken research for, or been a consultant to, several hearing aid and tinnitus device manufacturers.

APPENDIX I

Assistive Technology:
Secrets to Better Hearing

Working our way into the 21st century, the three most challenging listening situations are 1) understanding speech in noise, 2) hearing on the telephone, and 3) clarity of television. All of these can be effectively assisted through various amplifying devices, even in difficult and noisy acoustic environments. These *Assistive Listening Devices* (ALDs) essentially improve our connectivity to those we love and to sounds we enjoy and appreciate, like television and hearing on the telephone. What these benefits offer us at an emotional level is a restored connection to each other. The end result is not only improved hearing beyond hearing aids, but an improvement in your quality of life and everyone else around you. This auxiliary electronic equipment can amplify sound and enhance your ability to hear through the use of hearing aids as well as without them. The devices come in categories from amplified telephones to high intensity alerting equipment. As a result, your hearing experience is more pleasant, safer, requires less strain and frustration, and offers increased clarity and audibility. Any degree of hearing loss can typically benefit from these devices. If you have a hearing loss of even a mild degree, you can still benefit from many of these devices.

The primary connectivity pathway with current technology is through use of Bluetooth. This is a wireless (radio wave) connection to virtually any sound source. While Bluetooth itself is not actually built into hearing aids yet, there are "gateway" devices that permit benefit of Bluetooth. They function as a power source and control unit to integrate a Bluetooth signal from any sound source and convert it into a magnetic wireless signal that hearing aids process in real time. To explore what's available beyond the scope of this chapter, discuss your options with your hearing healthcare practitioner. Every top hearing aid manufacturer today offers these options in their hearing aids.

Some ALDs do not require that you even wear hearing aids in order to benefit from amplified sound such as television and some telephone. You'll find a wide variety of devices in this appendix that represent only a small sampling of what is actually available, from telephone and alerting products to television and signaling devices. Many of these devices actually solve hearing problems. Something as simple as not blasting the television (by having your own remote amplifier to your hearing aids) has solved many an argument and household disruption. You may want to contact ALD distributors directly (search them online) to broaden your perspective of what will best suite your hearing and financial needs. Some are referenced as you read through this appendix.

Most BTE hearing aids can accommodate what is called a Direct Audio Input (DAI). This system comes with a special manufacturer's designed boot (a coupler) that clips around your aid enabling you to plug into and listen to TV, radio, stereo, DVDs, FM or conference systems. Hearing aids that fit into the ear canal can also utilize direct audio input if they have the optional "T" switch on them. The DAI is a wonderful advantage to you because it offers the cleanest, clearest sound reception.

Your initial thought might be, "Why would I need DAI since I just purchased a top-of-the-line set of hearing aids?" Hearing aids are designed to amplify human speech, so you may derive added benefits from them (e.g., hearing the car radio better, or a dog whining to go out, but they may not adequately amplify specific auditory needs such as television, a doorbell or telephone ringing from another room.

Something worth mentioning is that not all hearing care practitioners carry ALDs in their offices. In a busy office many providers may feel ALDs are a distraction to their primary clinical functions. Don't be dismayed. Ask your hearing care practitioner for names of companies you can directly contact

Because wireless communication (such as cell phones) has come into being as a viable and important avenue of communication, this appendix includes cell phone devices that enhance your ability to hear. However, it's worth mentioning that cell phone designs have not really kept up with the personal needs of people with hearing loss, but it's improving. Technology changes quickly, so it's worth your exploration.

Names of companies cited as providing a photo courtesy of their organization is done to allow hearing healthcare professionals who might not be familiar with these devices and companies to have an opportunity on your behalf to contact them and establish an in-house corner of their office to display some hardware. Be cognizant of the warranty coverage you have on particular products. Some items carry only a one-year warranty while others have five years. Some companies have no fees for returns while others may charge you a restocking fee. Make these inquiries before you make the purchase.

DISCLAIMER: *Listing of products should in no way be construed as an endorsement of any company, product or device by the Publisher, the Editor or any contributing authors in this book. Any purchases of these devices are a responsibility between the reader and the company from which the purchase is made. Also bear in mind that these products were not rated in any way. That is, it cannot be assumed that a particular product listed in this Appendix is any better or worse than a comparable item available elsewhere.*

Typical Hearing Aid Challenges

- background noise
- reverberation (echo)
- distances between you and the person talking

Benefits of Assistive Technologies

- not all assistive technologies require your hearing aid
- acoustic feedback can be eliminated
- loudness may be increased
- low cost to buy
- easy to operate
- improves sound quality
- standard in most hearing aids (usually half shell or larger)

Bluetooth Requirements

- You'll need a T-coil in the hearing aid.
- The greater your hearing loss the more powerful will be the Bluetooth requirement of the T-coil. (Some tiny completely-in-the-canal hearing aids requiring minimal power can be utilized.)
- An optional Direct Audio Input (DAI) connects to the hearing aid and sends audio signals (e.g., radio or television) directly to your hearing aids by means of very high quality transmission when the power from your neckloop is insufficient. (You can request this from your hearing care practitioner.)

Loop Systems

"Looping" is a process whereby a T-coil carries the transmission of a high quality signal through an assistive listening device (ALD) or hearing aids. This is discussed in Chapter Twelve by Dr. Myers. Through use of your own hearing aids by switching the instrument to the T-coil mode, you can enjoy whatever sound source is looped.

Many movie theaters and houses of worship are now looped. Some hearing healthcare practitioners sell and install these loops; others work with local contractors who can install a loop system in your home.

Television
[FM / Closed Caption / Infrared]

An FM listening system makes TV very easy to hear. You can listen to multiple sounds using your personal FM system, so long as it is hooked up with a patch cord that goes from the audio output jack from the sound source into the auxiliary input found on most personal FM receivers. A personal FM system consists of one transmitter, one receiver and accessories. If you have a particularly significant hearing challenge, you might even consider using this system with closed caption.

Closed Caption is the ability to read printed text of dialog on the bottom of the TV screen generated from programs on television. You might have noticed on your TV remote control the letters CC. If so, your TV can utilize closed caption. If your TV was manufactured after 1993 and has a 13" or larger screen, it has this capability. If your TV doesn't have closed captions, you can purchase a decoder.

Infrared (IR) receivers and transmitters work well for television listening with smaller hearing aids or through headphones. The IR transmitter rests on top of the TV, and when not in use, the stethoscope-style IR receiver is stored in its battery charger. This is usually accomplished by means of a neckloop. A magnetic field moves through the loop to make it a fully wireless FM system. Then it sends an invisible signal to the hearing aid T-coils. For those who have a weak T-coil because you have an unusually small hearing aid in your ear canal (versus a behind-the-ear style), the solution might simply be raising the neckloop closer to your hearing aids. If that doesn't work, you might purchase a single or dual "silhouette" to provide a stronger signal.

Infrared Television Products

There are a few manufacturers who make television amplification systems. Some of these can be used with your hearing aids; others without. Three companies are listed on the following page. Figure A-1 represents what any of these devices essentially look like and how they basically operate.

TV Ears 5.0 Dual Digital Wireless Infrared System has excellent Voice Clarification Circuitry® to clarify dialog and a stethoscope-style receiver for mild to severe hearing loss with volume that can be set up to 120 dB (Figure A-1). Because of its power, caution should be taken regarding your listening level. One TV Ears transmitter can manage multiple headsets. It requires a three-hour charge and is rated for up to six hours of use on a full charge. This TV Ears system is compatible with any model television, old or new.

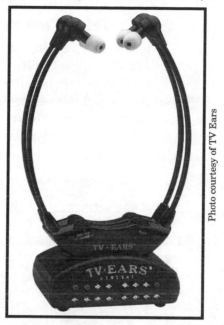

Figure A-1: TV Ears rechargeable infrared earphones

Sennheiser Direct Ear 100—IR TV Viewer (formerly AudioLink) operates and hooks up like TV Ears. It's slightly more expensive than TV Ears because it has a tiny screwdriver adjustment for volume and tone for each ear that may be important to you. Direct Ear offers optional microphones and additional headset receivers.

Sennheiser's Set 810S is another option for TV Listening system. It has an IR transmitter which recharges the batteries overnight and a round receiver/volume control that clips onto your clothing. It can be used with your own headset and no hearing aids. Should you choose to use it with your hearing aid T-coils, you should consider purchasing the Audex™ stereo neckloop (AD-NL-16.)

Williams Sound WIR 238 makes a small area stereo IR system with a stethoset receiver (2.3 MHz/2.8 MHz). It's ideal for TV listening, meetings or small group listening applications where you set the volume to your comfort without disturbing others in the room. The system connects directly to your TV or other devices with standard output jacks and has angled ear couplings for comfort and performance. An On/Off switch is built into the receiver so it can never be left on to drain the batteries.

Enhanced Listening Systems

Pocketalker Pro has easy-to-reach volume and tone controls, is reliable, modestly priced and shipped with an omni (multi-directional) microphone, a 12-foot mic extension cord for use with TV, and your choice of couplers: headphones or earbuds (Figure A-2). Two AA batteries provide about 100 hours of life. Additional options to consider include a three-foot cord, a neckloop, and to help reduce background noise it has a directional microphone.

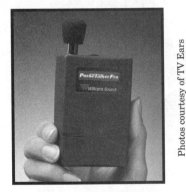

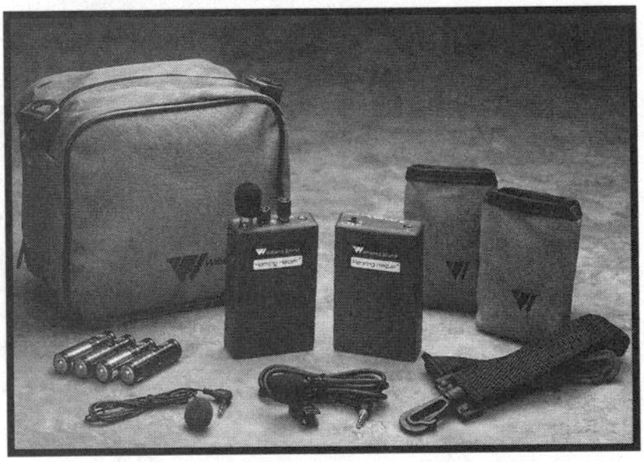

Figure A-2: PockeTalker Pro™
for common listening needs

Figure A-3: Hearing Helper™
for conference listening needs

Hearing Helper Personal FM System (FM350E) is a wireless multi-function system (Figure A-3) that transmits up to 150 feet. It's good for classrooms when the sound source is further away. You can add an R-31 receiver and its T-31 companion transmitter along with additional receivers to benefit multiple listeners. For cost savings, the R-31 receiver can be used with an inexpensive Y-cord (y-shaped cord to both ears of an ALD) and two directional lapel mics when around noise. Another option is the LA277 Conference Microphone with single or dual mic for improved hearing around a table. It's an inconspicuous two-inch triangle that plugs into the FM transmitter.

Amplified Telephones and Accessories

Although many younger and middle age people seemed to have moved to cell phone usage for their primary telecommunications, many older folks have been slower in this transition. Desk phones still remain in many homes. For those preferring and still using these telephones, you should know that most states have a free loan program and a variety of phone-related accessories for eligible residents so long as you have an "audiologist certified" letter indicating need. A quick online search can reveal a variety of amplified telephones that will meet most hearing needs and budgets. Some practitioners carry amplified phones in their office and allow you to take them home to try them prior to purchasing. If you buy online, note your degree of hearing loss (in dB) so you can correctly identify the appropriate phone for you.

Caption Telephones now make it remarkably easy to hear as well as read conversation in real time. If you are certified hard of hearing, the FCC will provide your choice of a free caption telephone. There are a few competing companies that sell similar products. One telephone might have larger number pads while another is styled as a more typical telephone. In the same way as captioned television works, caption telephones print the text of the conversation on a screen portion of the telephone—even on a cell phone that has Internet capability and a good screen on which to read captions. Figure A-4 shows one example of a desk phone with captions. No special equipment is required and it's free anywhere in the US that is Wi-Fi enabled, such as in coffee shops and hotels.

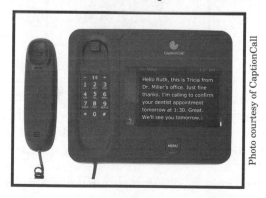

Figure A-4: CaptionCall uses customizable audio settings to match an individual's unique hearing loss while utilizing voice-recognition technology to caption conversation onto a large easy-to-read screen

Some choices for caption companies include:

- www.CapTel.com
  [They provide captioned and amplified telephones.]
  (800) 233-9130
  Email: captel@captel.com
- www.CaptionCall.com
  [They provide captioned and amplified telephones.]
  (877) 557-2227
  Email: support@captioncall.com
- www.HamiltonCaptel.com
  [They provide apps to visualize text for cell phones.]
  (877) 455-4227
  Email: info@hamiltoncaptel.com

Clarity XL-C3.5 is a cordless telephone that can be used without hearing aids, but with an audio output jack on the side of the phone, you can hear using both ears (Figure A-5). A stereo adapter plug is available for the jack that accommodates a neckloop, silhouette or cochlear implant adaptor cord. This system provides up to 50 dB of amplification, comes with tone control and 1 year warranty.

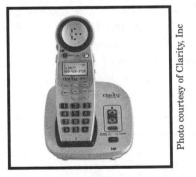

Figure A-5: Clarity XL-C3.5 maximizes power with adjustable volume

Serene Innovations VM-150 Answering Machine is one example of an amplified answering machine for those with hearing loss when you need to hear messages. It has up to 40 dB amplification, 22-minutes of recording time, remote access, and battery back-up.

Serene Innovations PA-30 Portable Phone Amplifier is only a few inches square and allows you to amplify telephone conversation up to 26 dB (and fits in your pocket). Merely strap it to the receiver portion of any telephone. It operates on 2 AAA batteries.

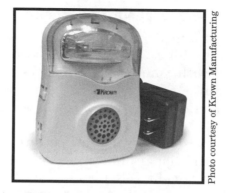

Figure A-6: **Krown Amplified Ringer** is a loud incoming ring signaler

Krown Amplified Ringer will catch your attention for incoming telephone calls with its blaring audible signal and bright strobe light that flashes (Figure A-6). This is for people with significant hearing loss because it blasts a 120 dB signal as well as the bright flashes. Caution should be taken if people in the house have normal hearing, since you don't want to risk causing hearing loss to anyone.

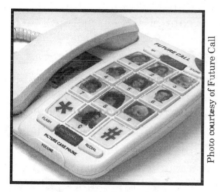

Figure A-7: FC-Picphone with photo touch screens

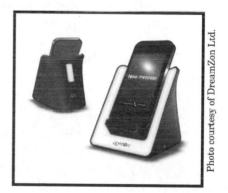

Figure A-8: DreamZon LightOn™ Cell Phone Signaler

FC-Picphone allows up to 10 oversized photo buttons for one-touch speed dialing (Figure A-7). It has up to 40 dB amplification, handset volume control, a loud adjustable ringer with flashing lights, desk or wall mount, and requires no phone cord or batteries.

DreamZon LightOn Cell Phone Signaler is a cradle that holds your cell phone. It will notify you of an incoming call with a bright LED pattern after it senses the vibration in your cell phone (Figure A-8). No plugs or installation and uses only 3 AA batteries (included).

Some about Cell Phones

Whether you use a modern smart phone or an older flip phone, the most important thing you can do is discuss your cell phone accessory options with your hearing healthcare provider. These products essentially eliminate hearing aid feedback, which has historically been a serious barrier to pleasant and effective telephone use.

You might also consider visiting the website of your hearing aid manufacturer for additional information and see what else they might offer you to benefit cell phone use. All top hearing aid manufacturers have a website and usually represent accessory products for cell phones.

You will also want to explore all options of amplified cell phones with your cell phone store. Before you make the purchase, you can even ask for an in-store trial so you can test if the amplification meets your needs. For invaluable information and a better understanding of cell phone technologies, access "Cell Phones Decoded" authored by Samuel R. Atcherson, PhD. and Patricia Highley, AuD., published in *Hearing Health* magazine and available on the Internet at http://online.qmags.com/HH0413#pg1&mode2.

Helpful Telephone Accessories

There are a variety of ear pads, cushions and devices available online by searching for your specific needs. For example, you can search for "listening pads" or "Bluetooth accessories / hearing aids." The cushioned (sponge-like) products ring the receiver and seal in the hearing aid to reduce and even eliminate acoustic feedback on a desk-type style telephone. Since there's no direct audio input, the greater your hearing loss, the greater the risk for feedback. However, Bluetooth capability for cell phone-type telephones eliminates the air waves by means of direct audio input and is the best way to fully eliminate acoustic feedback and enjoy conversation.

Alerting and Signaling Devices

There are a variety of fully-functioning alert and signaling devices for hard of hearing people. These include doorbell, intercom, baby cry signalers, and visual signalers that control a table lamp or even room lighting. These visual indicators can also be wirelessly connected to smoke and fire alarms, and some are easily portable for use in other places when you travel.

Alarm Clocks

Serene Innovations VA3 Travel Clock will awaken you by a powerful audible alarm (adjustable), vibration, or both (Figure A-9). It has tone control, a large bright easy-to-read screen, and a built-in flashlight, timer and thermometer for room temperature display. Included are a pillow clip and 3 AA batteries, along with a 1-year manufacturer's warranty.

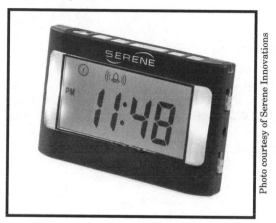

Figure A-9: Serene Innovations VA3 Travel Clock

Sonic Shaker SBP100 is an easy-to-read bedside alarm clock compact enough for safe travel in its own case (Figure A-10). It has a built-in powerful bed shaker and a 90 dB pulsating alarm. The clock has a 4-minute snooze, adjustable swivel and bright LED numbers for easy viewing. It comes with one AAA and two AA batteries, along with a 1-year manufacturer's warranty.

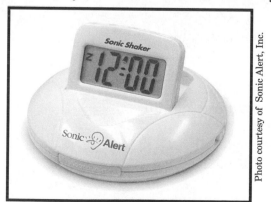

Figure A-10: Sonic Shaker SBP100 Alarm Clock

Resources for Assistive Technology Products

Adco Hearing Products
800-726-0851
www.adcohearing.com

Clear Sounds Communication
800-965-9043
www.clearsounds.com

General Technologies
800-328-6684
www.devices4less.com

Global Assistive Devices
888-778-4237
www.globalassistive.com

Harc Mercantile
800-445-9968
www.harc.com

Harris Communication
800-825-6758
www.harriscomm.com

Hearing Resources
800-531-2139
www.earlink.com

Hitec Group International
800-288-8303
www.hitec.com

Weitbrecht Communications, Inc.
800-233-9130
www.weitbrecht.com

APPENDIX II

Professional Resources

This Fourth Edition is fully updated to 2014 with relevant service organizations that offer information to anyone with hearing loss. Some offer leaflets or brochures and others offer referral services. Some don't have any current consumer services, but are listed here to allow you to write to them regarding questions you might have about a particular problem that you feel is best served by their group. Hopefully, this will give you the opportunity to expand your present search and gain additional knowledge.

These organizations may be reached by telephone, mail or email (if available). Keep in mind emails often change, but you can go to the website to obtain the current email contact. All of the groups listed have websites, so if you're Internet savvy, you can access them. In the text that follows, background, company function/mission, and their publications are included. If you write them for information, I encourage you to enclose a self-addressed return stamped (business-size) envelope, large enough to accommodate your requested literature. If you're telephoning, keep in mind that many of these offices are in the east (E.S.T. zone) and some close by 4:00 p.m.

Academy of Dispensing Audiologists

3008 Millwood Avenue, Columbia, SC 29205
Toll Free: (800) 445-8629
Email: info@audiologist.org   Website: audiologist.org

Founded in 1977, the Academy supports audiologists who dispense hearing aids. They must have achieved a graduate degree in the field, and in the near future, the only acceptable degree for membership qualification will be a doctorate. The Academy holds an annual meeting in the fall, and during the year smaller regional meetings and seminars providing information regarding all aspects of hearing aid dispensing. *Feedback* is their quarterly magazine for professionals that addresses topics and current issues pertinent to audiologists dispensing hearing aids. As of this writing, they are not staffed for consumer outreach although they offer consumer brochures and professional referrals to a practitioner in your local area.

Alexander Graham Bell Association for the Deaf

3417 Volta Place NW, Washington, D.C. 20007-2770
Voice: (202) 337-5220   TTY: (202) 337-5221
Email: info@agbell.org   Website: agbell.org

The Association is a nonprofit organization comprised of individuals who are hearing impaired, and their parents, professionals, and others. The organization's mission is to empower those with loss of hearing to function independently by promoting universal rights and optimal opportunities. They provide scholarships and awards to students and their families. They publish two periodicals, one research based, the other consumer oriented. There are over 20 chapters in North America, all of which provide leaflets on a range of problems affecting those suffering with hearing loss.

American Academy of Audiology

11730 Plaza America Drive, Suite 300 Reston, VA 20190
Toll Free: (800) 222-2336   Voice: (703) 790-8466
Email: info@audiology.org   Website: audiology.org

The Academy is a professional membership organization of audiologists. They have two primary journal publications. *Audiology Today* is a magazine format that deals with a wide variety of topics including clinical activities and hearing research. The *Journal of the American Academy of Audiology* publishes scientific papers of a scholarly nature. The Academy provides audiologists with current practice information and ongoing research knowledge. Their annual national meeting allows clinicians and scientists a forum for exchange and education in the areas of hearing science and hearing aids. They are not staffed for consumer outreach although they offer consumer brochures and professional referrals.

American Academy of Otolaryngology
—Head and Neck Surgery, Inc.

1650 Diagonal Road, Alexandria, VA 22314-2857
Voice: (703) 836-4444   Website: entnet.org

Founded in 1896 as a medical specialty society, they now have 11,000 physician members who provide medical care and surgery for disorders of the ears, nose, throat, head and neck regions. The primary missions of the Academy are to provide continuing medical education and to represent the interests of the specialty in governmental areas. The Academy publishes about a dozen patient education leaflets on various aspects of hearing loss which are available to the public at no charge. They also will refer you to a local practitioner if you specifically request the "Physicians List."

American Speech-Language-Hearing Association
10801 Rockville Pike, Rockville, Maryland 20852
Toll Free: (800) 638-8255   Voice: 301-296-5650
Email: actioncenter@asha.org   Website: asha.org

ASHA is a national professional and scientific association for audiologists and speech-language pathologists. Their mission is to ensure that all people with speech, language or hearing disorders have access to quality services to help them communicate more effectively. They inform the public about communicative disorders through published materials available by request. They can also provide professional referrals.

American Tinnitus Association
P.O. Box 5, Portland, OR 97207-0005
Toll Free: (800) 634 8978   Voice: (503) 248-9985
Email: tinnitus@ata.org   Website: ata.org

The ATA exists to cure tinnitus through the development of resources that advance tinnitus research. Founded in 1971, ATA has raised and allocated millions of dollars toward medical research projects focused on a cure. They also advocate for public policies that support its mission. ATA publishes a triannual journal written for a nonmedical audience including detailed articles on current research, treatment and other information for those living with tinnitus and others interested in staying current on this field of research.

Better Hearing Institute
1444 I Street NW, Suite 700, Washington, DC 20005
Toll Free: (800) 327-9355   Voice: (202) 449-1100
Email: mail@betterhearing.org   Website: betterhearing.org

BHI, a nonprofit educational organization, implements public information programs on hearing loss and available hearing solutions for millions with uncorrected hearing loss. The Institute promotes awareness of hearing loss and help through television, radio, and print media public service messages that typically feature well known celebrities who themselves suffer from impaired hearing. You may contact them for literature on hearing loss or specific subjects such as tinnitus, hearing aids, children's ear conditions, lists of local hearing professionals, and assistive listening devices. You or friends can also take their online hearing check at www.hearing check.org.

Hearing Education and Awareness for Rockers [HEAR]

San Francisco Center on Deafness

P.O. Box 460847, San Francisco, CA 94146
Voice: (415) 409-3277   Email:hear@hearnet.com   Website: hearnet.com

HEAR is a nonprofit public-benefit health organization founded in 1988 by Kathy Peck and Flash Gordon, M.D. They inspired large numbers of musicians and medically concerned physicians, music lovers and other music professionals to participate with them. Their advisory board consists of some members—now hearing impaired—from a variety of the loudest 1960's Rock 'n Roll bands. The organization is dedicated to raising consumer awareness about the risks of noise, and its damaging effects on hearing. They achieve this through television and radio public service messages featuring well known artists. Also, they have outreach programs which distribute hearing information and earplugs at music concerts/conferences, health fairs and community events. You may contact them for a free leaflet about noise risks. They've also produced a video on this subject for use in schools.

Hearing Health Foundation

363 Seventh Avenue, 10th Floor, New York, New York 10001-3904
Toll Free Voice: (866) 454-3924   Direct: (212) 257-6140   Toll Free TTY: (888) 435-6104
Email: info@hearinghealthfoundation.org
Website: hearinghealthfoundation.org

This foundation dates back to 1958 (under different names and ownerships). It has awarded many research grants that have improved treatments for otitis media, otosclerosis and cochlear implants. You may subscribe to their free quarterly publication,

Hearing Health Magazine, to keep informed of the latest discoveries that donations help make possible. Articles range from technological research and development, to humor, human success stories, and philosophical discussions about topics like education, cochlear implants, modes of communication, and living without hearing.

Hearing Loss Association of America

7910 Woodmont Avenue, Suite 1200, Bethesda, MD 20814
Voice/TTY: (301) 657-2248   Email: info@hearingloss.org
Website: hearingloss.org

Hearing Loss Association of America is the nation's foremost consumer organization representing people with hearing loss. HLAA impacts accessibility, public policy, research, public awareness, and service delivery related to hearing loss on a national and global level. Their national support network includes an office in the Washington D.C. area, 14 state organizations, and about 200 local chapters. Their mission is to open the world of communication for people with hearing loss through information, education, advocacy and support. They provide cutting edge information to consumers, policymakers, business professionals and family members through their website publications *Hearing Loss* (an online newsletter) and *ENews* (their message board). In addition, they bring consumers and policymakers together to learn about hearing accessibility issues at their national and regional conventions.

International Hearing Society

16880 Middlebelt Rd., Suite 4, Livonia, MI 48154
Toll Free: (800) 521-5247   Voice: (734) 522-7200
Website: ihsinfo.org

The IHS began in 1951 as the primary organization for hearing aid dispensers. They conduct programs of competence qualification and training, and offer continuing education courses in the selection, fitting, counseling, and dispensing of hearing instruments. They also publish an industry quarterly magazine, *The Hearing Professional*, articles of which cover industry news, membership highlights and best practices, hearing healthcare legislation, and other information and tools for hearing healthcare professionals. For a dispenser in your area, you may contact them.

Center for Hearing and Communication—NY

50 Broadway, 6th Floor, New York, NY 10004
Voice: (917) 305-7700   TTY (917) 305-7999

Center for Hearing and Communication—Florida

2900 West Cypress Creek Road, Ft. Lauderdale, FL 33309
Voice: (954) 601-1930   TTY: (954) 601-1938
Email: info@chchearing.org   Website: www.chchearing.org

CHC is a not-for-profit agency specializing in hearing rehabilitation and human services for infants, children and adults who are hard of hearing, deaf or deaf-blind. They offer support to recipients in their struggles to gain communication and other access in places of public accommodation, the workplace, and government facilities.

National Institute on Aging - Information Center

31 Center Drive, Bldg. 31, Room 5C27, MSC 2292, Bethesda, MD
20892-2292
Toll Free (800) 222-2225   TTY: (800) 222-4225
Email: niaic@nia.nih.gov   Website: nia.nih.gov

The NIA is responsible for the conduct and support of biomedical, social, and behavioral research, training, health information dissemination, and other programs with respect to the aging process and the diseases and other special problems and needs of the aged. They publish a number of detailed leaflets on aging.

National Institute on Deafness and Other Communication Disorders [NIDCD] - Information Clearinghouse

31 Center Drive, MSC 2320, Bethesda, MD 20892-2320
Toll Free: (800) 241-1044
Voice: (301) 496-7243   TTY: (800) 241-1055
Email: nidcdinfo@nidcd.nih.gov   Website: nidcd.nih.gov

This is a branch of the U.S. Government's National Institutes of Health. They're a clearinghouse that provide information on hearing, balance, smell, taste, voice, speech and language disorders, and develop and distribute publications that include fact sheets, bibliographies, information packets and directories of information resources. The Clearinghouse also publishes a biannual newsletter.

Index